SOCIAL ASPECTS OF CLINICAL MEDICINE

Social Aspects of Clinical Medicine

JESSIE GARRAD
B.A., B.Sc., A.I.M.S.W.
Lecturer, Department of Clinical Epidemiology and Social Medicine
St. Thomas's Hospital Medical School, London
formerly Senior Medical Social Worker
University College Hospital, London

and

Professor Sir MAX ROSENHEIM
K.B.E., M.A., M.D., P.R.C.P.
Director of the Medical Unit
University College Hospital Medical School, London

London
Baillière Tindall and Cassell

First Published 1970

7–8 Henrietta St., London W.C.2.

ISBN 0 7020 0340 9

Published in the United States of America
by the Williams & Wilkins Company, Baltimore

Made and printed in Great Britain by
Cox and Wyman Ltd., London, Fakenham and Reading

CONTENTS

ACKNOWLEDGEMENTS

We are most deeply grateful to Dr. Harold Lambert, Physician to St. George's Hospital, who, as Senior Medical Registrar, was for some years associated with us at University College Hospital. His was a major role in the lengthy preliminary discussions that led us to write this book and its emergence in its present form owes much to his enthusiasm and encouragement and to his valuable constructive criticism.

We would have liked to express our thanks to the many individual members of the senior staff of several hospitals and to the general practitioners who have kindly allowed us to quote problems and case reports, but for the sake of their patients' anonymity they must themselves remain anonymous. We have, over the years, learnt a great deal from the nursing staff, students, housemen and registrars who took so active a part in discussions on social problems and we hope that this book may ease the way for their successors.

Special thanks are due to Dr. A. E. Bennett, of St. Thomas's Hospital Medical School, for most helpful advice on problems related to occupation in Chapter 3. We also wish to thank Miss F. M. Picken, librarian at St. George's Hospital Medical School, for production of the index and Mrs. M. Rowe, Mrs. S. Kaye and Miss S. A. Smeeton for secretarial assistance.

But before I treat a patient . . .
I need to know a great deal more about him,
Than the patient himself can always tell me.
Indeed, it is often the case that my patients
Are only pieces of a total situation
Which I have to explore. The single patient
Who is ill by himself, is rather the exception.

T. S. ELIOT
The Cocktail Party

INTRODUCTION

It has long been customary on the Medical Unit at University College Hospital Medical School to hold 'Social Medicine Conferences' at which a student gives an account of one of his patients, emphasising the social problems that have emerged. These problems, which may be concerned with the aetiology of the patient's condition or may be interfering with his total care, are then discussed by the students, by the medical social worker, by the doctors and the ward sisters.

These conferences have proved both interesting and instructive, but often discussion of the individual patient has had to give way to an explanation of available social services and of the differing approaches that may be necessary to local authorities or voluntary bodies. Many years ago one of us produced a small pamphlet that outlined the various medical and social services available in the Welfare State and the present book has grown out of this as a result of discussions between the Medical Social Worker, the then Senior Medical Registrar to the Medical Unit and the Professor of Medicine.

The discipline of Social or Community Medicine implies an understanding of the social structure of the community and of the epidemiological and statistical techniques that may be used for investigating disease in the community. It also involves a knowledge of ways in which disease with social causes may be alleviated and the social causes minimised. This book is not concerned primarily with the community, but with the individual patient in his relation to the community in which he lives. The social aspects of clinical practice are becoming increasingly important and whether the young graduate is to become a general practitioner or to remain in the hospital service, he must inevitably need to recognise social aspects of disease and to understand how he can help his patients by invoking the many social agencies that are now available and anxious to help.

Increasingly in the future the clinician will be the leader of a team, a team that will comprise at least the medical, nursing and social services, and free communication between professions and free use of available services will help his patients and lighten the doctor's own personal responsibility.

Each patient differs in his genetic background, in his upbringing, in the environment in which he lives and works and in the social and emotional factors that may have played a part in precipitating disease and which must modify the effects of his disease and his reaction to it. Appreciation of the existence of such factors is essential if the doctor is to provide the optimum help for his patient. One of the great attractions of clinical medicine lies in the doctor–patient relationship, the interplay of personalities, and it is often only when a bond of confidence has been established that many of the social factors affecting the patient's condition may be revealed.

Illness can no longer be regarded as an isolated incident to be treated in a hospital bed or consulting room without reference to the environment. Medical students today are keenly aware of the importance of social and psychological stresses at play in the community and can readily appreciate their potential effect on their patients. Hospital personnel are becoming increasingly aware of the role of true 'district hospitals' with responsibility for the health of a defined community and recognise the need for close cooperation with the general practitioners and local authorities; while the individual doctor is increasingly concerned with the social, environmental and emotional problems of his patients and with the realisation that teamwork is going to be required for their full relief.

The efficient and most economic utilisation of all the available medical and social services is impaired by the present tripartite structure of the National Health Service with the general practitioner service, the local authority services and the hospitals. It is widely accepted that some unification of the medical services is required. This was proposed by the Porritt Committee and has recently been suggested in the form of Area Boards by the Green Paper while the report of the Seebohm Committee recommends changes in the local authority personal social services. As this book goes to press all these recommendations are under discussion. Changes in the organisation and control of medical and social services appear likely. As these may lead to changes in the procedure for seeking aid, the availability of existing services may be improved, but the provision of additional services is largely dependent on the investment of additional resources.

The aim of this book is, therefore, first to present the patient as an individual in the community and to review those social, environmental and emotional factors that may play a part in his disease, and secondly to examine the means by which the community services can be enlisted in his aid. It has, therefore, been written from the viewpoint of the practising clinician and, while making no claims to be a book on public health or on epidemiology, or a textbook of psychology, medical sociology or social administration, these disciplines have inevitably been invoked in outlining the relation of the patient to the community and the services offered by the community to the patient.

The first section of the book deals with the social history and reviews the various factors that must be considered and which may affect the patient or his relatives. This is followed by a series of case histories that illustrate the varied interaction between medical and social factors in disease with reference to the available sources of help. In the third section the medical and social services and their respective roles are considered and the need for free communication and cooperation is stressed. The final section summarises the medical and social services available and ends with references and suggestions for further reading.

This book has been written primarily to assist medical students during their early years in clinical medicine, but we hope that it may also prove of interest to the young doctor in hospital or in general practice, to nurses and to the growing team of social workers.

PART I

THE SOCIAL HISTORY: ITS CONTENT AND USE

1

THE PATIENT

The basic philosophy expressed in this book is that to provide a patient with the most appropriate medical care the clinician needs to consider the patient and his illness in his social setting. Many factors in his material and emotional environment may be relevant in the aetiology and treatment of his disease and it may be as important to identify and evaluate these as to note his physical signs and symptoms and his mental state. These factors can usually be identified by taking a careful social history. Like the medical history this is not best achieved by direct questioning since a more revealing history can be obtained if the patient can be prompted to talk about himself as he wishes, although with a verbose patient the course of the interview must be guided by the doctor. Valuable indications of the patient's personality and attitudes can be obtained from the way in which he describes his social situation while his order of priorities is often a useful pointer to the important factors and to his feelings about them.

As the patient's social history emerges the details should be catalogued mentally and ordered into 'systems' as in this way gaps in the information can be identified and the missing data obtained by judicious questioning. The social factors of potential importance in clinical medicine can usefully be considered, both in practice and for purposes of this discussion, under five 'systems' or headings: family, occupation, housing, finance, relationships and attitudes. Detailed information under each heading is not necessary in every case and, with increasing skill in recognising social factors relevant to medical conditions, it is possible to adapt the form of the social history to suit each patient.

When taking the history the doctor has an excellent opportunity to start to know his patient as an individual. At the same time the patient forms his first general impression of the doctor and realises that he is a person in whom he can place his confidence and trust and to whom he can talk freely. From this initial interaction develops the doctor–patient relationship which forms one of the bases of good medical practice (see Chapter 6). By his general manner and his comments the doctor should show that he accepts the patient as he is, without making value-judgements on his actions, his family relationships, his scale of values or any aspects of his life. This is of great importance when the patient's situation or actions are ones about which most people have their own strong feelings or opinions. If the doctor appears to sit in judgement or in other ways shows his own feelings he may prejudice the establishment of a good professional relationship. For example, an unmarried pregnant woman usually has some feelings of guilt at having transgressed the usually accepted moral code, whether or not she is fully aware of the feelings or whether she shows them by timidity or by apparent indifference. She will therefore be ready to interpret any impatience or abruptness from the doctor as a sign of disapproval and rejection and this may result in her defaulting from antenatal clinics or refusing needed help from a social worker. Whereas if the doctor shows concern for the medical and social welfare of herself and her child without indicating approval or disapproval of her action, he will help to establish a feeling of trust and security. If her first contact with a professional person is helpful and constructive this attitude of trust will probably carry over to the other professional workers to whom the doctor may refer her, such as a social worker, health visitor or midwife; this will increase the chances of achieving successful medical care and social resettlement of the patient and her baby.

The full social history may not be obtained at the first meeting of doctor and patient. The patient comes to discuss his symptoms and to seek relief. Relevant social details may only emerge with encouragement from the doctor after he has assessed the presenting problem and when the patient has got to know his doctor.

Details about a patient must be treated in confidence by the doctor but, with the development of the team approach, which is discussed in Chapters 8 and 9, this knowledge often has to be shared with a group of professional people. In order to provide appropriate medical and social care, administrative arrangements may require sharing of information with an increasing number of people in separate but allied organisations. This is acceptable provided the personnel have the same standards of professional confidence as the medical, nursing and social work professions; if, however, the information is to be handled by large numbers of untrained people, such arrangements may not always be in the patient's best interest. A safeguard, therefore, is to obtain the patient's consent before passing information about him. This is particularly important when an employer or solicitor asks for a medical report and in such cases it is always necessary to obtain consent in writing.

THE FAMILY

In most societies the family is the basic social group providing the individual with his material, emotional and cultural environment. Within this group the child first learns the use of language and concepts, establishes his first personal relationships, undergoes normal psychological development and learns the accepted forms of behaviour and the moral code. Cross-cultural studies show the wide variation in the cultural norm between people of different races and between different sub-groups and classes in a complex society. These variations are seen in the differences of family organisation and in the distribution of responsibility between the members of the family; in methods of child-rearing; in the warmth of emotional relationships; in the severity of discipline; and in the acceptable canons of behaviour. Disruption of one aspect of the typical pattern is often followed by changes in another. For example, in Great Britain behaviour that differs from the norm so much as to be unacceptable to society is more frequently shown by children from broken homes, where the parents are divorced or separated, than by children from homes where the parents are living happily together (see Chapter 6).

It is therefore important to obtain details about the patient's immediate family, its composition, the ages of the various members and particulars of their occupation or schooling and any relevant comments about their health. From this type of information several deductions can be made. First, it is possible to assess the patient's family responsibilities: for example, he may be a married man with several dependent schoolchildren and a wife unfit to work outside the home; or she may be a single woman living at home and helping to support and care for an elderly parent. Such information helps the doctor to appreciate the disruption caused to family life by illness and the patient's natural anxiety about it. Together with knowledge of the patient's prognosis, it enables the doctor to predict social difficulties likely to arise in the future, some of which he may be able to help the patient to anticipate and deal with. This forms a useful guide in the difficult task of deciding how much information about diagnosis and prognosis he must give the patient to enable him to make realistic decisions affecting himself and his family (see Case History No. 1).

Because of the ramifications of family life few patients can be treated in isolation and the sympathetic understanding and co-operation of other members is usually necessary (see Case Histories Nos. 1, 4, 8, 12, 14). From the social history one can get an indication of the availability of relatives who may be able to give additional information about the family medical history and about the onset of the patient's illness and who may be able to help in planning and furthering the patient's rehabilitation or care. From this and from his subsequent personal knowledge of the family, the doctor can decide who is the most suitable relative with whom to discuss the patient's diagnosis and prognosis, especially if it is considered inappropriate to discuss this with the patient himself.

If the patient is a child the social history is best taken from an adult member of the family although the child may be able to add his own, often revealing, comments. The social history will show whether his mother goes out to work and the extent to which she may be free to care for him in the future; it will show who looks after him in her absence, whether grandmother, neighbour or registered child-minder (see Case Histories Nos. 2 and 3).

It has been said that the relatives can be the doctor's greatest ally or his worst enemy. Relatives working with the doctor can aid not only the patient's physical progress but can also help to foster a forward-looking attitude; conversely they can hinder treatment either by indifference or lack of care or by over-protecting the patient instead of encouraging his independence within the limits of the illness.

This cooperation of the relatives has to be sought; they need to be shown in what ways they can help, and to do this well they need to know relevant details of the medical situation and its possible outcome. When giving information to the relatives (or to the patient) the doctor should avoid the use of technical terms unless he explains them first. In the medical setting, so many phrases become part of daily use and so many words acquire a specific connotation that it is easy for the doctor to forget that they are not part of current usage and that they may be unknown, or their specialised use misleading, to the layman. The information he gives and the way in which he presents it should be adjusted to the ability of the patient or relatives to understand it. In this way he will avoid talking over their heads or, equally undesirably, of talking down to them. Since the introduction in 1948 of comprehensive national insurance and a comprehensive medical service, doctors come into contact with a more representative selection of the population. This change has been further accentuated by improvements in the standard of living since the pre-war depression and in the general education of the population.

With the present popularity of medical topics in press, radio and television there is a greater awareness by all sections of the population of medical diagnoses and treatments and a correspondingly greater expectation that the doctor will discuss the relevant information with the patient and his relatives. However, although they want to be given this information, they are usually anxious and tense while being told and, as a result, often do not register or fully understand everything that is said, although the doctor may have given a simple and lucid explanation. It is therefore often necessary for him to repeat it on several occasions (see Case History No. 4). Time spent by the doctor in 'taking the relatives with him' is time well spent (see Case Histories Nos. 1, 2, 3, 9, 11, 12). It will help to reduce their anxiety, much of which often arises from not understanding what is happening; and anxious relatives make for anxious patients.

The general practitioner or family doctor is in the most advantageous position to establish this relationship with the relatives as he visits the patient's home and often maintains contact with the family over many years (see Case Histories Nos. 1, 7 and 13). In hospitals, this contact between doctor and family often goes by default especially when technical aspects of the hospital doctor's work are demanding and time consuming. It is the responsibility of the doctor to seek out the relatives and he should discourage attempts by the nursing staff to 'protect' him from them. The relatives have a right to see the doctor and the house officer should make a practice of seeing the responsible relative at each stage of the patient's illness; the chief should also be available when necessary. Too often in the past the only occasion when relatives saw a doctor in hospital was when they were asked to give permission for a postmortem.

When attending a hospital, a patient may see several doctors on the same or different firms as well as many non-medical personnel. When there is this team approach it is desirable that one doctor should be the formal channel of communication and responsible for ensuring that the members of the team, patient and relatives all know what is happening.

3

OCCUPATION

OCCUPATIONAL HAZARDS

Work in certain industries or trades carries a known risk of developing a specific or 'industrial disease'. For example, inhalation of silica-containing dusts whilst working in mines or foundries can cause fibrotic lung disease. Many substances used in industry are toxic, such as lead or cadmium, or chemicals such as aromatic hydrocarbons; some compounds are dangerous in that they increase the liability of the exposed worker to develop cancer, as in dye or rubber workers exposed to β-napthylamine who experience an abnormally high incidence of cancer of the bladder. Certain infectious diseases may occur in particular jobs, such as anthrax in workers handling hides or Weil's disease in sewer workers.

Environmental conditions of work may also have adverse effects on health. For example, where the noise level is over 85 decibels workers may suffer from permanent damage to their hearing. This was formerly called boiler-maker's deafness as it was first recognised amongst boiler-makers, smiths and braziers. A workman may be unaware of developing deafness until it is severe and his first complaint is often that he cannot carry on a conversation within a group of people. A hazard affecting vision is exposure to intense heat or radiation which may cause cataract. Decompression sickness or caisson disease may result from work such as underwater construction or engineering in which compressed air is employed. Rapid decompression at the end of the shift may lead to intravascular formation of nitrogen bubbles, with neurological and other severe sequelae.

Prescribed industrial diseases are those conditions recognised to be the result of occupational exposure to risk. A man shown to be suffering from one of these diseases is entitled to claim industrial injuries benefit under the national insurance provisions (see page 145). These social security benefits may be quite substantial: Case quotes the history of one patient who received £2 5*s*. 6*d*. per week and back payment of over £500 because, although he had developed the disease five years previously, he was only advised that he could claim after attending a specialist hospital. In addition, a man who considers that he has suffered as a result of his employment may have grounds for summoning his employer under common law if negligence has been a factor.

There is no doubt, therefore, that it is in a patient's direct interest that his doctor should have a knowledge of industrial disease and be aware of all the implications of a patient's present or past occupations.

Apart from hazards to health from industrial exposure to toxic materials or adverse environmental conditions, more general aspects of a man's work may have some effect. Morris has demonstrated that workers who are physically active suffer less severely from ischaemic heart disease than sedentary workers, comparing bus conductors with bus drivers and postmen with male telephonists. However, caution must be exercised in interpreting such evidence as he has also shown that there are personal factors operating in self-selection for the different kinds of work, as bus drivers were heavier with larger physical measurements than the conductors when they took up the job. The commonly held belief that executives suffer more from duodenal ulcer seems to have little basis in fact. Studies by Dunn and Cobb in America have shown that the experience of foremen and chargehands is considerably worse than the senior executives' for this condition. However, comparison of morbidity and mortality in different jobs may be misleading: there may be different physical and psychological characteristics which lead men to select different jobs and these, rather than the job, may influence morbidity and mortality.

Knowledge of a patient's occupation therefore enables the

clinician to know whether he has been exposed to a particular occupational risk; whether he is a member of an 'at-risk' group. Consideration of a patient's illness in relation to the morbidity and mortality experience of his occupational group may thus give a useful pointer to a possible diagnosis. However, knowledge of the present or last occupation is not always sufficient as some of these diseases only become manifest a number of years after the man has left the industry, so a full occupational history may be necessary.

The occupational history is also of value in psychiatric assessment. Stresses at work are often important in provoking symptoms and it is relevant to know to what extent a patient's work corresponds with his interests, intelligence, education and capabilities: his relationships with other employees and superiors are also relevant. A history of very frequent and unaccountable changes of employment is common in patients of schizoid or psychopathic personality. As this kind of restless changing from job to job not uncommonly precedes a schizophrenic breakdown, a sudden change in the occupational history from steady employment to rapid job-change enables the start of breakdown to be identified.

USE IN AFTER-CARE

Knowledge of a man's occupation is essential when considering his after-care. Chronic disabling illness or accident may render a man permanently unfit to resume his usual occupation but leave him capable of doing another which is compatible with his disability. For example, a clerk of works having had a severe coronary thrombosis would be unfit to continue his job if his supervisory work involved climbing or working at heights, but he could continue satisfactorily if it consisted of administrative or physically non-exacting duties. Similarly an epileptic, even if his fits are controlled, needs special consideration and should not, of course, drive motor vehicles and it is desirable that he should not operate or work near moving machinery.

Considerable knowledge of the requirements of a job are necessary before a doctor can give a man advice whether he should change his occupation. The recommendation to change should never be made lightly as not only may the man's livelihood be at stake but his whole way of life and that of his family. In some cases the issues are clear-cut and the decision is obvious: in others a trial period on the job may show whether it is possible or wise to continue: in other cases he may be able to return to his own job in a modified form or to another job which requires the same skills but does not include that element which is incompatible with his medical condition. Only very occasionally is a definite change of employment necessary. When a job has to be modified or a change made cooperation with the man's employers is usually helpful, especially if there is a works' medical officer. However, before any approach may be made it is absolutely essential that the patient's permission is obtained in order to preserve the confidential professional relationship (see Case History No. 5).

In practice there are often difficulties when a man changes to another type of work. The alternative work that he can manage within the limits of his disability may be less skilled or less responsible than his usual job: this may be a blow to his pride and a further threat to his security which has already been shaken by the need to change jobs. In addition less skilled or less responsible work is usually less well paid, so he probably suffers loss of income as well as loss of status. In some trades, such as printing, the annual number of entrants is limited by trade union regulations and a change of trade or movement from one job to another within the same trade often requires the prior approval of trade union officials.

If a man's employer is unwilling or unable to offer suitably modified or alternative employment, the man has to give or be given notice of termination of employment. It is popularly supposed that an employer cannot end a man's employment during sickness absence but this is a misconception. For the most part employers are considerate and, if they have to replace a man during sickness absence, will often wait until after the worst of his illness before doing so. Since July 1964 when the Contract of Employment Act 1963 became operative, every employer is required to give each employee a written contract of terms and conditions of employment. This Act also states the minimum period of notice of termination of employment required by either party. At least one week's notice is required from an employer after a period of continuous service of 26 weeks or more: at least two weeks after two years or more: at least four weeks after five years or more.

When a man becomes unfit for his usual work through residual disability there are several ways in which the doctor and patient can receive informed advice about suitable vacancies with other employers or about alternative types of employment, including particulars of industrial rehabilitation and retraining courses (see Case History No. 6. Also see Part IV. Employment. Page 143).

CLASSIFICATION OF OCCUPATIONS

PRINCIPLES OF CLASSIFICATION

The grading of occupations into social classes was first attempted in 1911 by Dr. T. H. C. Stevenson of the General Register Office. He devised the classification which first appeared in the Census of England and Wales 1911 and which has been used as the basis of many subsequent analyses. His concepts and classification have since been tested by many sociologists and social psychologists. By compiling lists of different occupations to be ranked for status by a variety of people, children, adolescents and adults of varying educational levels and from different backgrounds, they showed that there was wide public recognition of occupational status and furthermore a remarkably consistent assessment of the status of a wide range of occupations.

CURRENT CLASSIFICATION

For the classification of the Sample Census of England and Wales in 1966, the General Register Office uses three stages. All industry is divided into 24 groups based on the nature of the industry or service. For example, group I comprises agriculture, forestry, fishing: group II mining and quarrying: and group XV paper, printing and publishing. The second stage of classification is the grouping of occupations within each industry for the purpose of providing 'groups with at least one common characteristic. The basic common factor of all groups is the kind of work done and the nature of the operation performed'. By this means all occupations are divided in 211 groups and these are then combined into a smaller number of groups based on the status of the occupation.

The most widely used grouping developed in this way is the Social Class Classification with the following divisions:

I	Professional occupations.
II	Managerial and 'minor' professional occupations.
III NM	Skilled non-manual occupations.
III M	Skilled manual occupations.
IV	Semi-skilled manual occupations.
V	Unskilled manual occupations.

This classification, which divides the entire working population into only six groups, obviously has defects but it is a useful tool, as differences in social characteristics between the groups are in general greater than the differences between occupations within the same group.

Another method of classification is by Socio-Economic Group and takes into account a man's status within his occupation, e.g. whether he is a foreman, supervisor or director. The aim is 'that each socio-economic group should contain people whose social, cultural and recreational standards and behaviour are similar'. In this classification there are 17 divisions and this partly overcomes the criticisms of the social class classification. It enables a finer classification to be made which is more revealing of differences: the five large groups of the social class classification tend to mask small differences. However, for some studies the social class classification is still preferable as it is an overall hierarchical scale while the socio-economic group classification consits of a number of sub-hierarchies.

SOCIAL CLASS PATTERNS OF DISEASE

It has been shown that workers in certain occupations are at risk of developing specific disease: they may be considered to be an 'at-risk' group. This concept may be applied more widely to different groups in the population. Comparison of disease prevalence or death rates in the different social classes may reveal significant variations. For example, some studies have shown that chronic respiratory disease is more prevalent in the lower social classes. This may reflect differences in smoking habits as well as differences in exposure to air pollution. Male mortality from lung cancer and stomach cancer is highest in social class V. By contrast, mortality of men from ischaemic heart disease and cerebro-vascular disease is highest in social class I. For females, the prevalence and mortality for cervical cancer is highest in social class V. However, for mortality from cancer of the uterus, excluding cervix, there is no detectable social class gradient. The finding of a social class gradient in disease prevalence or mortality strongly suggests that environmental factors are associated in the aetiology of the condition.

Social class differences may be studied over periods of time. During the last thirty years there has been a marked drop in the infant mortality rate for all classes but the social class differences still remain. This implies that the factors responsible for the differences between the classes have not been eliminated by modern health and welfare provisions. However, a degree of caution is necessary in examining changes over a period of time because the characteristics of groups based on an occupational classification do not necessarily remain the same. Similarly, social class patterns of disease in one country may not be found in another because again the social and economic characteristics may not be comparable. Nevertheless, in spite of the limitations of these classifications and the caution with which any findings are interpreted, they are valuable tools for studies of the population.

4

FINANCE

NEED FOR DATA

Closely associated with the patient's occupation or that of members of his family is the question of family finances.

Sickness may cause immediate financial hardship. In general, workers who are paid by the hour ('wage earners') are less often paid by the employer during absence through sickness than are employees paid weekly or monthly ('salaried staff'), who usually receive the whole or part of their salary for the number of weeks stipulated in their terms of employment. Small firms may not have such formal arrangements about sick pay and in these cases an ex-gratia payment is often made which is dependent on the employee's length of service and on the personalities involved. A report published in July 1964 by the then Ministry of Pensions and National Insurance showed the extent to which employees were covered by occupational sick pay schemes and described the provisions of the schemes during the year ending June 2nd 1962 (*Scope and Characteristics of Employers' Sick Pay Schemes*, H.M.S.O.). Such schemes covered 56·6 per cent of men, 52·5 per cent of married women and 62·3 per cent of single women. There was considerable variation in the qualifying period of employment and the duration of payment and there was a 'dramatic decline in the coverage and treatment with social class and occupational status'.

In addition to sick pay schemes there are also many private sickness clubs, such as the Hospital Savings Association, and forms of private sickness insurance such as the British United

Provident Association. Members or insurers pay a regular contribution which may range from a few pence each week to many pounds a year and this entitles them to various categories of cash benefit payments. Then there is the sickness benefit paid to a contributor with allowances for his dependants under the National Insurance Act 1946 and the industrial injuries benefit payable under the Industrial Injuries Insurance Act 1946 in cases of industrial injury or prescribed disease contracted during employment (for further details see page 145).

In Great Britain a patient need not incur high expenditure on medical treatment unless he chooses to be treated outside the National Health Service. A man normally resident in this country, or a bona fide visitor suddenly taken ill, is entitled to medical treatment which is 'free' in the sense that no payment is made at the time of treatment. A standard contribution is required towards the cost of prescriptions of outpatients and for some appliances but this can be reduced in cases of hardship (for details see page 127). National schemes of insurance and medical treatment are also well developed in several countries, for example Scandinavia, Australia and New Zealand. Great Britain has reciprocal arrangements with some of these countries whereby nationals of one country are eligible for benefit in the other. This is in contrast to some other countries, such as the United States, where the costs of treatment are extremely high and private insurance against illness is the rule for those who can afford the premiums, as the 'Medicare' provisions apply to selected groups of elderly people only.

Although in this country a man may not have high additional expenditure in time of illness, it has been shown that his income may be very different from normal and a consideration of family budgeting may be useful in certain cases (see Case History No. 5). When considering family budgeting the total family income should be roughly calculated on a weekly or monthly basis and against this should be set regular expenditure such as rent, rates, mortgage, insurance, hire-purchase payments (on articles ranging from clothes to cars), cost of heating, lighting and food. Full details are not needed in every case and when it does appear relevant it is desirable to give some explanation to the patient as to why the information is wanted. This avoids the charge of prying. When taking a social history it is wise not to ask for a piece of information unless good reason could be given if the patient were to challenge the doctor as to its relevance.

USE OF DATA

This information gives a guide to the patient's general standard of living, to his degree of nutrition and his material environment. It has been said that the treatment that is actually prescribed for a patient is often a compromise between what is medically desirable and what is socially possible: some knowledge of the patient's socio-economic status helps the doctor to judge whether his medical recommendations are realistic in the patient's situation. For example, in theory, most special diets do not cost more than a good balanced diet. However, many people are unable to afford a balanced diet and make up the bulk by eating cheaper foods containing a high proportion of carbohydrate such as bread and potatoes, and include little fresh fruit. For such people, a diabetic or gastric diet involves a great change in their eating habits and the purchase of more expensive foods. Also, if the patient is the only member of his family on such a diet the relative cost of his food will be even higher, as the cost of buying and preparing food for one is always higher than the cost per head of the same food prepared for a number of people. This is recognised by the Department of Social Security (formerly the National Assistance Board) whose officers are able to make an extra dietary allowance for people in receipt of a general allowance (see page 146).

The information may also throw some light on the patient's scale of values which may be relevant to his general medical management. For example, the middle class spend a high proportion of their income on food, housing and education. Many wage earners, whose weekly income may well exceed that of some professional people, spend a smaller proportion on housing and education but often have very high hire-purchase commitments and with the sudden drop in income through illness may, for example, pay for the hire of the television set before paying the rent. Illness may therefore result in debt and the re-allocation of limited funds according to the patient's order of priorities.

5

HOUSING

With most patients it is desirable to have some indication of their accommodation but with patients suffering from certain diseases or on certain treatments full details are necessary. These can be considered under a number of sub-headings.

LOCATION

The location is important especially in patients attending hospital as they often have to travel a considerable distance. It is often necessary to know whether they live in a town or in the country: if in a town whether in the centre or in the suburbs, in an industrial or residential area: if in the country whether in a small town or village, whether on a bus route or whether isolated from public transport. It is helpful to know whether the patient lives of a council estate or one in private ownership and whether it is a new estate occupied by young couples with children or an old estate with an established community of several generations. This type of information gives some indication of the characteristics of the community from which the patient comes, of the accessibility of his home and of the possibility of help from neighbours.

TYPE

The type of accommodation should be described, whether a house, bungalow, maisonette, flat or rooms. It is necessary to define the terms flat and maisonette as their usage is changing. Two or three rooms sub-let in a large house with the use of a shared lavatory, often on another floor, is now frequently referred to as a flat. However, the term is more usually used to describe accommodation consisting of a number of rooms, lavatory (with or without bathroom) and kitchen all on the same floor and forming a self-contained unit with a front door separating it from the rest of the building. Such accommodation is also sometimes referred to as a maisonette, although this term is usually reserved for self-contained accommodation on two or more floors forming part of a larger building.

It may be necessary to know whcther the property is owned or rented by the patient: if the latter, whether the owner is a local authority, a housing association or a private landlord, and whether it is let furnished or unfurnished. These factors are relevant if structural alterations or adaptations are necessary to meet the patient's physical needs, and also because they help to determine his legal position in the complicated legislation affecting the rights and duties of landlord and tenant.

CONDITION

It may be useful to know whether the premises are in good repair or whether, for example, the roof leaks or the lift is not working.

LAYOUT

Having determined the location and type of accommodation, the layout must be considered. First, which floor or floors the patient occupies. It is worth remembering that many patients refer to the ground floor as the first floor: that the hall floor in a nineteenth-century house is not at ground level being usually above a basement or semi-basement and reached from street level by a flight of steep stone steps, often with a low balustrade but no handrail. Then it is necessary to know the number and uses of the rooms, their spatial relation to each other, to the lavatory and water supply and to the stairs or lift.

AMENITIES

The amenities should be considered. First the type of sanitation is important, whether there is a flush lavatory in the house or in an out-house in the back yard, or whether there is outside chemical sanitation: whether the lavatory is used by the patient and his family only or shared by other families. Second, the water supply: whether, for example, this consists of a cold water tap in the back yard shared by all the families in the building, whether it is a sink and cold water tap on the landing shared by the families occupying rooms on that floor, whether there is hot water in the kitchen, whether there is a bathroom. Facilities for heating water may range from a kettle over a gas-ring to piped hot water in blocks of modern centrally heated flats. Third, the method of space heating should be noted: central heating, oil burners, electric, gas or coal fires and if the latter where the coal is stored. Fourth, whether the lighting is by electricity, gas or oil. Fifth, food storage and facilities for cooking are important and these range from fully equipped modern kitchens to a gas-ring in a bed-sitting-room. In this connection, the difficulty of preparing a special diet with very limited cooking facilities should not be overlooked.

USE OF DATA IN TREATMENT

These details are needed when considering the daily routine of patients with physical disabilities, such as those resulting from the rheumatic diseases, neurological conditions affecting the locomotor system, cardiovascular disorders or failing sight in elderly people. It is clear that certain housing conditions may provide practical obstacles to a patient's social rehabilitation (see Case Histories Nos. 4, 7 and 9). Some of these difficulties may be overcome by structural alterations, adaptations and improvements in facilities, as well as by the provision of 'gadgets'. This is one of the responsibilities of the local welfare authority (see page 128). These conditions similarly affect the care of patients needing nursing at home (see Case Histories Nos. 4 and 7). It may be necessary to arrange the loan of nursing equipment, such as a commode or bed-pan for a patient unable to reach the lavatory and to ensure that a relative, neighbour or home help is available to empty it for him. In some areas a cooked midday meal can be delivered to an elderly or disabled patient unable, through a combination of disability and inadequate cooking facilities, to prepare it for himself (see Case Histories Nos. 8 and 14). The advice of the health visitor is invaluable to doctor, patient and relatives when planning the home nursing of a patient, especially during a chronic or terminal illness. (See Chapters 8, 10 and 11 for a description of the health visitor's training and function.)

USE OF DATA IN DIAGNOSIS

While some aspects of the accommodation may cause difficulties in the rehabilitation or home care of a patient, others may be a contributory factor in the development of anxiety, depression or psychosomatic disorders, or behaviour difficulties in children. When this occurs it is usually because some factor in the situation is causing excessive emotional stress which the individual is unable to tolerate. This usually happens in one of four ways. First, overcrowding with the resulting lack of privacy creates tensions between members of a family and intensifies pre-existing strains. Minor disagreements become major quarrels when there is no space for the different generations to spend some time separately and difficulties arise when teenage children, sometimes of different sexes, have to sleep in the same room as their parents.

Second, if a family is living in an old building in poor condition the housewife usually suffers most. The rooms are difficult to keep clean, the necessity to carry water up and downstairs and lack of space to dry napkins and clothes makes household tasks an unrewarding struggle.

Third, disagreements with other tenants is a frequent source of unhappiness, particularly when water supply, cooking facilities or lavatory are shared by several families. The causes of friction range from complaints about children's behaviour to objections to the whole way of life of people from a different culture.

Fourth, disagreements between landlord and tenant can be a

major cause of anxiety, and requests for advice on these problems form the second largest category of enquiry received by the Citizens' Advice Bureaux (see page 103). In their biennial report for 1962–4 the National Committee state that about one quarter of the one and a quarter million enquiries brought to the Bureaux during the two and a half years covered by the report concerned some aspect of housing. For people renting accommodation in privately owned buildings the fear of being given notice to quit is a very real one and may prevent a tenant from making justifiable complaints to the landlord, for example, about the need for repairs or about the behaviour of other tenants. But a tenant occupying unfurnished property at a controlled rent, and therefore often referred to as a 'controlled tenant', has security of tenure subject to certain specified exceptions such as the tenant being in arrears with his rent or the landlord needing the premises for his own personal use. (Controlled rents are those for tenancies which began before July 5th 1957 in property that on November 7th 1956 had a rateable value of £40 or less in London and £30 or under in other parts of England and Wales.) The landlord can only regain possession if he can convince a Magistrate's Court that one of the specified conditions applies and if he can satisfy the court that he has offered suitable alternative accommodation to the tenant. Therefore a few unscrupulous landlords make the tenant's life intolerable in the hope that he will voluntarily move, leaving the accommodation available for letting at a decontrolled and much higher rent. Methods used range from delay in effecting repairs, especially to the roof and plumbing, to the letting of other parts of the building to tenants whose behaviour is unacceptable to the controlled tenant. Other methods of intimidation have been reported in the press.

A patient may therefore have good grounds for attributing his illness or delayed recovery to some aspect of his living conditions. However, there is a tendency for people to 'use' an illness in this way in order to enlist the doctor's support for their application for rehousing by a local housing authority. Such support should only be given if careful investigation shows the patient's application to be justified. This is not always the case: sometimes a patient will want to establish a link between his accommodation and his illness when the aetiology and treatment are unaffected by the physical environment. In other cases the position is more subtle. At the present time it is respectable to complain about housing conditions: such a complaint enlists the hearer's sympathy and demonstrates the speaker's wish to improve his circumstances: this is acceptable to society. For this reason, a complaint of housing difficulties is often used as a cover for other, less acceptable problems. As already shown, poor housing conditions may accentuate pre-existing emotional difficulties which may be a more fundamental cause of the illness: for example patients with marital difficulties often attribute their illness to housing problems. Such cases need very careful investigation and it may be that the patient would be better helped by the Marriage Guidance Council than by the local housing authority (see Case History No. 10). This case shows the difficulty of apportioning responsibility for illness when the patient is subjected to both material and emotional stress. Following their comments on housing, the National Committee of the Citizens' Advice Bureaux state: 'Approximately one further quarter of the enquiries relate to family and personal problems but bureaux workers point out the difficulties sometimes encountered of separating these two categories since bad housing may cause family disturbance, and family disturbance may cause bad budgeting, arrears of rent or eviction.' (Report 1962–64.)

Many trained personnel are available to assist the doctor in his investigation and treatment of such problems and by experience he will find the most appropriate for a particular patient. If the problem appears to centre round the need for structural repair the public health authority (see Chapter 8) will make a report to the doctor and require the landlord to effect the necessary repairs but, as shown below, this may sometimes have undesirable repercussions. If the doctor considers that the patient or housewife is not making the best use of the premises or managing the care of the family in the most appropriate way, particularly if young children, sick or elderly people are concerned, he can ask the health visitor to offer her services to the family (see Chapters 8 and 11). When the difficulties appear to be mainly due to faulty personal relationships the doctor may ask a trained social worker to offer help to the family. This is the type of medical social problem with which the medical social worker and the psychiatric social worker are specially trained to help (see pages 94–99 and 108). The problem of personal relationships, especially within the family as it affects illness, is considered in more detail in Chapter 6 (see also Case Histories 3, 7, 12, 13, 14).

The emotional stress caused by neighbours or landlords is often hard and sometimes impossible to alleviate. It is unwise for the doctor to take sides or give legal advice but the patient can obtain much advice through his own solicitor, or one participating in the Assisted Person's Legal Aid Scheme, or through a Citizens' Advice Bureau. Sometimes an informal approach by one of these people is sufficient to improve the situation. Legal action such as summoning the neighbour for nuisance or reporting the landlord to the public health authority who may summon him under public health and housing legislation often helps, but it may result in a vindictive retaliation and a worsening of the situation.

Sometimes the ideal solution would be the rehousing of the patient but with the present national shortage of accommodation at moderate rents the only realistic policy in most cases is to help the patient to make the best use of what he has. The local housing authority provides accommodation at subsidised rents but as demand far exceeds supply most authorities have some system of assessing the relative priority of each would-be tenant and medical factors are only one of many taken into consideration. To augment this service, the local housing authorities are empowered by the Minister of Housing to offer mortgages on favourable terms to encourage house purchase, to make improvement or discretionary grants for the modernisation or conversion of old property and to assist the formation of housing associations under which groups of families buy, convert or build accommodation on a non profit-making, joint-ownership basis. (For details of local housing authorities see page 118 and page 147.)

6

ATTITUDES AND RELATIONSHIPS

CULTURAL ATTITUDES TO ILLNESS

'There is no reason why the social data should not be of the same scientific value as those from the laboratory or X-ray department. The time is gone when we had to content ourselves with information on the composition of the family, number of rooms, rent and sleeping arrangements, and the questionable presence of a bath, when asking about the social conditions of our patient. We know now that in order to understand the patient we must learn about his family relations, ties and tensions, his work, friends, aspirations, hopes and frustrations, about his development, his attitude to his place in society, his habits, his compensating and escape mechanisms.' (Querido).

In the preceding chapters we have shown the importance of appreciating the patient's relationships with his family and those with whom he works and relaxes. In this chapter we consider the patient's attitudes and in particular his feelings about illness and his relationships with those treating him and we attempt to demonstrate their importance in clinical medicine.

The sick person is always regarded as different from the fit person but attitudes towards him vary in different cultures. It has been suggested that in western industrial societies there are four characteristics of the sick role (Parsons):

(a) The sick person is exempt from his normal duties and responsibilities in proportion to the nature and severity of his illness.

(b) It is recognised that his illness is 'legitimate' and that he cannot just 'pull himself together' so he needs to be taken care of. It follows from these attitudes that

(c) the sick person has an obligation to 'get well'.

(d) The exemption from responsibilities and the provision of care depend on this response from the sick person and the conditional nature of these privileges are a defence by society against malingering.

In order to get well the sick person is expected to seek the help of a professional expert, the doctor, and to cooperate with him in treatment. Thus an ill person may be told that he 'ought' to see a doctor, that he 'ought' to be in bed. Therefore when a person is ill, the community gives him certain privileges provided he takes appropriate action in order to resume his usual place in the community as soon as possible. It has been suggested that, while in America illness is seen primarily as a threat to the achievement of the individual, in Great Britain it is seen as a threat to his status as an acceptable member of society (Parsons, 1958). The emphasis in treatment is therefore on reintegration into the community. Consequently the individual is thought to have a 'right' to treatment which will lead to his reintegration and to his resumption of his responsibilities in and to the community. This philosophy leads to the acceptance of the principles of a national health service. By contrast, in America, the threat to the achievement of status of an individual is considered to be a personal matter and therefore it is up to the sick person to pay for the professional expertise that will assist him to resume his activities. In Great Britain, somatic illness is accepted by the community as being beyond the individual's responsibility, he cannot 'help' being ill. Mental illness is still not always regarded in this way and is therefore less readily tolerated although professional and popular attitudes are changing.

When the sick person becomes a patient by seeking a doctor's services, three special features of his situation become evident. He is in need of help but he cannot define what help is necessary: he cannot assess the doctor's technical competence therefore he does not know whether he is being given the appropriate help and he is thus put in a position of dependence: thirdly, he is emotionally involved in the situation (Parsons 1951). His illness cuts him off from his usual activities and disrupts his social relationships; he may be humiliated by his inability to function normally and by his dependence on others and the more independent he usually is the harder will this be to accept. He may have to bear discomfort or pain and to face the frustration of his ambitions and, in some cases, the possibility of death. Therefore at the start of an illness, the patient is often in a state of emotional shock and later he may develop anxiety about the future. This is very clearly seen in men who have suffered a coronary thrombosis: often there is shock at the suddenness of the episode, fear of the pain and great apprehension for their survival: this is often followed after an interval by intense anxiety about their future prognosis, their work prospects and ability to resume their usual way of life.

In the role of the medical practitioner four characteristics can be discerned (Parsons, 1951): (a) It is a sub-group of the larger group of professional occupational roles but one which has become functionally specialised for caring for the sick. The high level of technical competence necessary to fulfil this function has resulted in long and specialised training followed by the award of publicly-recognised authorisation to practice. (b) However, the high level of technical competence is restricted to the field of medical practice and does not confer authority in other fields. (c) As in applied science, the medical practitioner's role involves an affective neutrality. He is expected to assess all evidence 'objectively': he is required by the mores of his profession and by the community to treat all patients to the best of his ability regardless of their status and whether he likes them as people. (d) Finally, the medical practitioner is expected, again both by the mores of his profession and the community, to put the welfare of his patient before his own personal interests.

The acceptance of these responsibilities by the medical practitioner enables the community to accord him certain 'privileges'. Many facts relevant to diagnosis or treatment are topics which the patient would not normally discuss except with intimates, even if with them. However, it is generally accepted that a doctor may need this confidential information. In all communities there are accepted standards controlling the amounts and occasions of bodily exposure and contact. Again it is accepted that it may be essential for a doctor to see and examine a patient's body and the community modifies the usual behavioural code accordingly.

INTERACTION OF DOCTOR AND PATIENT

It has been shown that the roles of doctor and patient respectively carry recognised responsibilities and privileges which are largely complementary. Three main types of interaction between doctor and patient have been described (Bloom). In the activity-passivity relationship, the doctor is the active member of the pair and the patient is passive and accepting of treatment: this situation exists when the patient is unconscious or too ill to make much response. In the guidance-cooperation relationship, the doctor makes recommendations to the patient and encourages cooperation by giving explanation and appropriate information (see Case Histories Nos. 5 and 9). This is the most usual form of relationship especially in cases of acute illness. In the situation of mutual participation, the patient is accepted as a partner in the medical care process, although less informed, and alternative courses of action are jointly discussed and the most appropriate selected for implementation. This approach is often adopted in cases of chronic illness where the patient has learned to live with his disease and understands many of its implications (see Case Histories Nos. 1 and 6). These three classes of relationship show a gradient in the activity of the patient *vis-à-vis* the doctor. The ability of the patient to assume one of these relationships depends not only on the nature and severity of his illness but on his age, intelligence and ability to express his thoughts and feelings in words. It depends also on his temperament and on his concept of the doctor's role and of his own as a patient. The doctor's ability to encourage or tolerate the patient's response depends on his temperamental preference for an authoritarian or permissive approach and on his perception of the patient's abilities, needs and preferences.

These three types of relationship are not discrete categories but rather three points on a continuum as the doctor-patient relationship is a dynamic, continually changing interaction. The same doctor may establish a different type of relationship with one patient than with another and with the same patient at different stages in the illness, the nature of the relationship depending on the factors already described. This change is also clearly seen in the case of a patient with a coronary thrombosis. Immediately after the episode, the doctor may need to take active life-saving measures on a relatively inactive patient. Later during the acute phase of fear, the patient needs firm reassurance and clear-cut instructions about his regime and some explanation of what has happened to him. Later, when he is worried about his long-term prospects, he benefits from informed discussion of his prognosis and working ability. At this stage doctor and patient may agree that he should return to his old job for a trial period and both would assess his progress.

The delicate balance of this relationship is influenced by other cultural and emotional factors. The majority of patients have less education and come from a lower social class than the majority of doctors, the professional group being the smallest in the population. The 'middle' classes use a larger vocabulary and appreciate more abstract concepts than do the 'working' class. They also use a form of language in which the nature of the words and their order in the sentence convey nuances of meaning and expression of emotion which are not readily understood by working class families (Bernstein). In addition, the form of language that an individual uses greatly influences his modes of observation, perception and interpretation in all aspects of life (Saphir). These cultural differences can easily limit understanding between patient and doctor and adversely influence their relationship unless the doctor, having greater verbal facility, adapts his language-use to that of the patient. In addition to these cultural differences, the doctor uses a professional medical vocabulary largely unknown to the majority of patients and it is essential to explain these terms, if they are used at all, when talking to patients and relatives so that misunderstandings may be avoided.

Among emotional factors, the attitudes of doctor and patient are important in the professional relationship and these also are influenced by cultural factors. The doctor and patient may have a different scale of values and the doctor needs to recognise this and to understand the patient's attitudes in order to make appropriate recommendations. For example, members of the medical profession naturally place a high value on health and consider that much should be sacrificed to attain it. For example, a general practitioner in a northern industrial town advised some of his patients with early chronic bronchitis to move to an area with less air pollution in order to lessen their chances of deterioration but few acted on his recommendation (Susser and Watson). The doctor placed a high value on health and was a member of the professions who expect to move home to take up alternative employment. By contrast, his patients were from the lower social classes who generally expect to remain in their homes and to find alternative employment locally. (This is one of the reasons why the Department of Productivity aims to establish alternative industries in areas of high unemployment and so move the work to the workers.) The value that the patients placed on health was not sufficiently great to overcome their cultural preference for remaining in their home district.

PERSONAL ATTITUDES TO ILLNESS

In addition to differences in values, the doctor and patient may have a different attitude towards the patient's illness. The doctor has been trained to assess the situation objectively, to recognise his emotional response and to limit its effect on his judgement as far as possible. The patient, however, is suffering, he is intensely involved in the situation and he may have much at stake. To bridge this gap, the doctor needs to appreciate what the illness means to the patient in terms of social disruption and also its psychological significance. Illness involves some measure of dependence. It may be dependence on the doctor's professional expertise in order to regain one's health: it may be continued physical and emotional dependence on relatives and many professional people. To the person who is normally very independent physically and emotionally, dependence constitutes a serious threat to his personal integrity and this will be manifest in his behaviour to the doctor and others and in his response to treatment (Storr) (see Case Histories Nos. 4, 7 and 14).

Similarly, a particular illness may have a different significance to doctor and patient. The doctor has knowledge of the cause, natural history and treatment of an illness: the patient may have no knowledge or such as he has may be incomplete and inaccurate. For example, a doctor knows that certain cancers can be treated and have a high survival rate: to most laymen cancer is a lethal disease and anything the doctor may say to a patient or relative may be interpreted in the light of this belief. Also, the patient's previous experience of illness, either personally or in others, will influence his attitudes, his response to illness and hence affect his relationship with the doctor (see Case Histories Nos. 4, 9 and 12). The meaning of the illness to the patient may be elucidated if the doctor can answer the question 'Why has *this* patient come to me with *this* illness at *this* time?' (Balint).

CULTURAL FACTORS AFFECTING ILLNESS

Among the peoples of developing countries, health education programmes and the provision of preventive and therapeutic medical services similar to those of western industrial countries are often given an ambivalent reception. The traditional systems of care express cultural attitudes to illness and treatment which are not easily reconciled with those of western medicine. It has been shown that it is necessary to understand the cultural values and beliefs that control traditional health practices and dietary traditions in order to establish communication and influence entrenched attitudes (Read). When treating immigrant people in this country it is necessary to be aware that their attitudes to illness and treatment may be very different from those of the indigenous population, while second-generation immigrants born and bred in this country may be in a transitional stage. Bloom quotes the case of a 55 year old American–Italian who had lived in America for forty years but who retained all the Italian cultural characteristics. She was a diabetic for whom insulin and a restricted carbohydrate diet were prescribed but the patient continually failed to follow her diet and exasperated her consultant. When transferred to another doctor, she was successful in keeping to her diet. In a careful analysis, Bloom shows that the early difficulties were primarily due to the first physician's failure to recognise that he and his patient held four different value-orientations. The American culture values individualism while Italians put the family before the individual, so that the patient would not risk upsetting the family's social pattern. The physician expected that his patient would sacrifice present pleasures of eating to achieve better health in the future while she lived fully in the present, accepting the future fatalistically. The physician believed that man could control nature, including illness, while the Italian peasant's attitude is that man is helpless. Finally, the physician in American culture is a 'doer' and expected his patient to be active also: but in Italian culture 'spontaneous emotional expression takes precedence over doing'.

Not only may differences in cultural attitudes and behaviour patterns have an adverse effect on treatment but they may be a cause of illness. There is some evidence that the incidence of mild psychological illness rises when a community is broken up by redevelopment programmes and the residents rehoused in new housing estates or in new towns. This is attributed to the loss of feelings of community, to the sense of not belonging, to the loss of support from older relatives and from the familiarity of neighbourhood customs.

Similar feelings of isolation may result from social as well as geographical mobility. During this century, greater educational opportunities have enabled many people to enter occupations barred to their parents. It has been shown (chapter 3) that a whole cluster of social characteristics are associated with occupation and social class and these have to be learned by the socially mobile. The period of transition may therefore be a time of stress which in turn may be a cause of illness.

The immigrant from overseas experiences in more extreme form the differences in culture and difficulties of adjustment that are experienced by the geographically and socially mobile in this country. The period of transition from one culture to another, the process of acculturation, is thus one of importance to the medical practitioner. The experience of social isolation, the feeling of not belonging, may also be found among people who are disfigured or disabled (Hunt) and there is some evidence that physically disabled people may show more psychological disturbance than the non-disabled. (Bennett and Garrad.)

These subjective feelings of social isolation may arise when a person's self-assessment, cultural values and ambitions are undervalued by the society in which he lives and when he is prevented, by whatever reason, from achieving the approval and acceptance of that society. It has been shown that the form of behaviour by which psychological disturbance is manifest depends on the culture in which the abnormal behaviour occurs. Thus, while there may be a genetic basis for the major psychoses and for some of the neuroses, the symptoms by which these become manifest will vary in different cultures (Linton). This kind of process may perhaps be detected in the current vogue for drug taking. In every generation people with psychopathic personalities and others experiencing social isolation have expressed their difficulties by deviant behaviour. During the last fifty years there have been many changes in the cultural patterns of this country particularly in the problems of child-rearing, in the behaviour of adolescents and in the status of women. (Carstairs.) Perhaps it is not surprising therefore that disturbed or isolated adolescents express their difficulties in a new way. The relative shortage of reliable information on the psychological processes of drug dependence and of the action of different drugs has increased public alarm at this new phenomenon. In terms of numbers the problem is thought to be small but in terms of personal unhappiness and family tragedy it is a serious and pressing problem.

It is thus necessary, when history taking and at all the later stages of caring for patients, to be aware of the varied and subtle ways in which their society and cultural background influence the attitudes of both doctor and patient and their relationship with each other.

PART II

RELATED MEDICAL AND SOCIAL FACTORS

7

SOME ILLUSTRATIVE CASE HISTORIES

In Part I we discussed the need to consider certain aspects of the patient's personality and social situation when making a diagnosis or deciding the most appropriate management. Although every patient is unique, the broad principles discussed can be applied in a wide variety of medical and social situations. In this part we describe a number of cases which illustrate how these principles may be implemented and we attempt to show how consideration of these factors in each case influenced decision-making.

CASE HISTORIES

1. THE MANAGEMENT OF TERMINAL ILLNESS

MEDICAL SITUATION

Mr. A, aged 52, was admitted to hospital for investigation and was found to have extensive carcinoma of the oesophagus with secondaries in the liver. A thoracotomy was performed and a Celestin tube inserted in the oesophagus. His prognosis was estimated at about six months.

SOCIAL SITUATION

Mr. A was married but had no children. His nephew, aged 22, who lived with him and whom he regarded as a son, had recently died from a cerebral embolus.

Mr. A had held a variety of jobs but for the last ten years had worked as a shop assistant. He said he earned 'good money', was being paid during sickness and had 'comfortable savings'. He had a self-contained, comfortably furnished flat in a block with a lift.

He and his wife were a devoted couple who recognised that their childlessness had drawn them closer together. They were good companions and each was fully in the other's confidence.

PROGRESS

On admission, Mr. A suspected that he had cancer and discussed with the medical social worker his fears of cancer and of surgery. His religious beliefs were a great support to him and he received much assistance from the hospital chaplain. He was not afraid of death, but of suffering. Post-operatively, because of his attitude, the surgeon agreed to his request to tell him, as well as his wife, the details of his diagnosis and prognosis and assured him that he would be kept free of pain. As soon as he knew the position, Mr. A became much calmer and started to plan for his wife's care following his death. He used the medical social worker as a 'sounding board' with whom he talked out alternative plans until he and his wife agreed on final arrangements.

PATIENT'S CARE

Mr A was insistent that he wanted to die at home and his wife, although apprehensive, agreed to meet his wishes. They both had great confidence in their general practitioner whom they, as well as the hospital staff, consulted about home care plans before his discharge. The medical social worker suggested to Mrs. A that her husband could be admitted to a small hospital for terminal care should his condition become too difficult for her to manage at home. On the advice of her general practitioner, she agreed to his name being put on the waiting list and the knowledge that such facilities existed reduced her anxiety over her responsibilities of home nursing. The general practitioner agreed to supervise the patient's home care and to give the wife all the support she needed.

About six weeks later, the general practitioner considered that Mr. A had developed cerebral secondaries and was too difficult for Mrs. A to continue nursing. He asked for a terminal care bed. When this was offered three days later Mr. A refused to be admitted. The general practitioner respected his patient's wishes and gave additional support to the wife and arranged for the district nurse to help her with the nursing until Mr. A died at home one week later.

POINTS TO NOTICE

1. The surgeon's use of his knowledge of the patient's character and attitudes in deciding what to tell him of his diagnosis and prognosis.
2. The key role of the general practitioner in the patient's management.
3. The general practitioner's respect for the wishes of his patient and wife and his cooperation in meeting them.
4. The patient's use of the medical social worker to relieve some of his anxieties about cancer and to help him to fulfil his responsibilities to his wife.
5. The comfort derived by the wife at knowing of the existence of a special hospital for terminal care.

2. A YOUNG FAMILY WITH MULTIPLE PROBLEMS

THE FAMILY

Bobby was six weeks old when he was first admitted to hospital with a feeding problem. His sisters were aged two and a half and one year. His mother was seventeen: his father was in his twenties and usually unemployed and living on supplementary benefit. The family occupied a flatlet in a homeless family unit administered by the local welfare authority.

THE MOTHER

The mother's parents had been separated for some time and she had never felt her own mother to be a person to whom she could look for support. At an early age she turned elsewhere for acceptance and at fourteen she was pregnant by the man she later married. She was a warmhearted girl and had retained an unsophisticated spontaneity and in spite of her early responsibilities seemed no older than her seventeen years.

THE FATHER

The father also came from a poorly functioning home which had left him with many fears and little assurance. His father had been an alcoholic and, although his parents had remained together, there had been much stress and as a boy he had been much neglected. He was now a rough and ready, workshy man lacking in confidence and afraid of authority.

THE MARRIAGE

As the father's sexual relations with the mother under the age of sixteen (the age of consent) was an offence in law, the couple had come under the care of the probation officer who had provided some stability, compensating somewhat for their unsatisfactory home backgrounds. The mother had also formed a helpful relationship with the medical social worker at the maternity hospital and with social workers of a Roman Catholic voluntary organisation when she had stayed in their mother and baby home for single girls. This social help, which had started before their marriage, enabled them to withstand the strains of their early relationship, strains which were both intrinsic in their personalities and due to practical problems, particularly of accommodation. Their own families had been unwilling or unable to share their homes with them so that eventually, being technically homeless, the young family was accommodated by the local welfare authority in a homeless family unit.

The birth of the second child had brought strain but the third child (the boy now in hospital), born within eleven months of the second, had brought intolerable stress. There had been violent scenes between the parents before the baby's admission and the young mother was tense with resentment. The aggressive behaviour, the lack of financial support, the quarrels, the resulting chaos at home had brought the family to the point of disintegration. When the baby was admitted the mother was seeking legal separation, the father had already withdrawn from the situation and their tenancy of the welfare authority flatlet was about to be terminated because of the general disorder and lack of cohesion in the family.

SUPPORTING THE FAMILY UNIT

The child care officer, the health visitor, the local N.S.P.C.C. officer and the homeless family welfare worker were all concerned with the family but in spite of close liaison between all of them and the hospital's medical social worker, discharge plans for the baby failed twice. After the first discharge the baby quickly deteriorated and was readmitted; only one day after his second discharge the mother applied to the child care officer for all the children to be taken into the care of the local authority children's department and placed in residential or foster homes as she could not cope with them. Her application was refused as being unconstructive. The baby became ill again and was admitted a third time together with the second child aged one, leaving the two and a half year old girl with the mother.

By this time, the family's tenancy of the flatlet had ceased and the mother and father were living apart in furnished rooms. However, they both visited the babies regularly and, in the protected environment of the hospital, they enjoyed being with their children and appeared to wish to be together. Through good hospital teamwork many departments cooperated in the family's rehabilitation. It was agreed to encourage the parents increasingly to take over the care of their children in hospital and a room in the hospital was set aside for the family. The ward sister played a large part and the medical social worker was needed. The dietician informally tried to demonstrate more adequate meal planning and preparation. Meanwhile the medical staff remained closely in touch not only with the young family but also with the other members of the hospital team.

This coordinated attention to their medical and social problems encouraged the young couple and it began to seem to them to be both possible and worthwhile to resume their responsibilities as parents together. The local welfare authority was persuaded to reallocate another homeless family flatlet. The mother wanted to discuss with the medical social worker what her difficulties were likely to be and how to plan to meet them. It was a delicate matter for the medical social worker to decide how far it was wise to offer help, either practical or advisory, and how far the responsibility should be left to the couple. Some financial help was obtained to meet practical needs but care was taken to let the mother decide for herself what were her main requirements. Within a short period the parents were enthusiastic to take over the care of all the children and, as the baby was then quite fit, the children's discharge was speedily arranged.

REFERRAL TO COMMUNITY WORKERS

The children did not then need medical follow-up from the hospital and it seemed desirable that further support, both social and medical, should be given by community workers. The child care officer had already visited the hospital and talked with the parents as well as the hospital staff and was fully aware of the medical and social situation; the general practitioner and health visitor were also informed. The hospital medical social worker made a final visit to see the family settled in their new flatlet and the community workers took over responsibility for continuing support. The young couple fully understood and accepted this.

POINTS TO NOTICE

1. The impossibility of satisfactorily treating the baby's medical condition without 'treating' the family's social difficulties.
2. The carefully coordinated help provided to the family by the different professional staff in the hospital.
3. The way in which the parents were helped to resume responsibility for the family themselves.
4. The close liaison between the hospital staff and the community workers.
5. This couple's practical and emotional problems were increased by having three babies in two and a half years. Unfortunately, it is often the couples who have the greatest need to space the pregnancies who do not seek advice on methods of contraception or who are unable to follow the instructions.

3. THE PROBLEMS OF A HANDICAPPED CHILD

THE BABY

Caroline was admitted to the ward at the age of one year with upper respiratory tract infection. She was a spastic with a severe right hemiplegia and was mentally retarded. She did not pull herself up nor sit up but lay in her cot rocking her body or head-rolling. However, she recognised her mother and showed that she welcomed her visits.

THE FAMILY

Her parents were not married. She had an elder brother aged two years and another of three weeks. Her father had been unemployed and finally left the family before the birth of the third baby. Her mother had therefore placed Caroline and her elder brother with a foster mother and had worked throughout her last pregnancy to support the family.

They lived in one rented, medium-sized furnished room in which they cooked, ate, washed and slept. When the mother stopped work at term, her allowance from the Department of Social Security was £3 5s. 6d. per week, plus the rent.

MOTHER'S ATTITUDE

Understandably, the mother was depressed and anxious. It was difficult to assess her feelings about Caroline's disability and her consort's desertion. She had an obvious sense of responsibility and she wanted the hospital staff to know of her social situation and her practical difficulties in order to explain why she had been unable to care adequately for Caroline. When she realised that her difficulties were fully appreciated she became more relaxed and less depressed and anxious.

DISCHARGE PLANS

The medical social worker discussed various alternative plans for Caroline's care with the mother, but the mother was aware of the value of her close relationship with Caroline during the baby's early years and she decided to take her home rather than put her in a residential nursery or mental deficiency hospital. She agreed to bring Caroline to the hospital twice a week for physiotherapy even though she would have to bring the other two children also, but she was relieved that she was still to keep in touch with the hospital staff. Her financial position was eased by an increase in her weekly allowance and by a grant from a voluntary benevolent fund. The general practitioner, the health visitor and the local authority mental welfare officer were informed of the situation and Caroline was discharged home.

OUTPATIENT FOLLOW-UP

The mother managed reasonably well during the next few weeks, and the visits to hospital gave the opportunity for continued support from the medical staff, physiotherapist and medical social worker. Her life, though busy, was lonely and she was glad to talk about her many difficulties. It transpired that while she was carrying Caroline there had been many quarrels and temporary separations between herself and her consort. When Caroline was born prematurely he rejected the handicapped baby and soon afterwards left home for the last time. By then the mother was again pregnant by him. The mother therefore associated Caroline's handicap and his desertion, and her emotional conflicts about him were reflected in her care of the little girl. When she became depressed, treatment lapsed and she became pessimistic about the child's future and her own responsibilities. During one of these phases Caroline again developed an upper respiratory tract infection and was readmitted. This time the mother's feelings were reflected in her failure to visit regularly. After three months of treatment, appropriate feeding and skilled care, Caroline developed considerably. Again her mother felt capable of caring for her at home and after a week or two of readjustment Caroline settled down happily at home where her mother was supported by the community workers.

Her mother continued to be isolated and lonely with heavy family responsibilities, but by the end of the year the youngest baby, the boy, was walking and the two most difficult years of Caroline's life were over. In more than the physical sense, she too was at last on her feet.

POINTS TO NOTICE

1. The mother's association of Caroline's handicap and her consort's desertion.

2. The way in which the mother's feelings influenced her management of the child.
3. The continued support needed by a 'fatherless family', particularly when there is the added problem of a handicapped child.
4. The impossibility of separating medical and social aspects in such situations.

4. A PATIENT WITH SUICIDAL TENDENCIES

MEDICAL SITUATION

Mr. D, aged 55, suffered from multiple sclerosis and was admitted to hospital following a suicide attempt by an overdose of barbiturates. The medical social worker's assessment suggested that a further attempt seemed likely so he was referred to the psychiatrist. (Such referral is now standard practice in all cases of attempted suicide.) He considered that a further attempt was likely in the absence of help but that psychiatric treatment was not needed provided the patient was given active social support. Mr. D and his wife were willing to cooperate in social rehabilitation plans.

SOCIAL HISTORY

Mr. D was a Pole who had left his Polish wife and son on the outbreak of war and since then had lived with a British woman by whom he had a daughter, aged 16.

He served with the Polish Merchant Navy as a stoker throughout the war and then transferred to the British Merchant Navy. He was discharged as medically unfit in the early 1950s and had been more or less unemployed since, living on sickness benefit and supplementary allowances. His wife, a former nurse, did not work and his daughter was an apprentice hairdresser. They occupied two ground-floor rooms with adjacent kitchen in a privately-owned nineteenth-century house with semi-basement. The daughter had one room for her bedroom while Mr. and Mrs. D. had a 'Put-u-up' in the sitting-room. The lavatory was on the first floor and the bathroom on the third floor, both shared with other tenants.

Mr. D was demonstrative in his affection for his 'wife', while she was taciturn but had considerable understanding and tolerance of his moods. They were very proud of their daughter whose welfare they put before their own.

At the time of admission Mr. D was emotionally labile but very depressed about his increasing disability. In his suicide note to his wife he explained that he did not wish to be a burden and wanted to free her and their daughter to live happily together. Two years previously he had attended the neurological department of another hospital; when he defaulted on an appointment and was not followed up by the staff he concluded that they could not help him. During his current admission he accepted that help was available but felt humiliated by his dependence on help for physical needs.

REHABILITATION

At the time of his admission Mr. D was able to dress himself with help for fastenings, to wash unaided at the kitchen sink, and to crawl on all fours to the first-floor lavatory where he needed assistance with his clothing. As an inpatient he attended the hospital's Aids to Daily Living Department, where an exact assessment was made of the nature and amount of help he needed with self-care (dressing, toilet, feeding) and which gadgets would increase his independence. He attended the physiotherapy and occupational therapy departments, first as an inpatient and then as an outpatient.

Long-term plans were also started. An application was made for him to attend the sheltered workshop run jointly by the local welfare authority and the Department of Employment and Productivity (formerly the Ministry of Labour) for people too disabled for competitive employment. A hand-propelled chair was ordered through the Department of Health to enable him to go out with his wife, and a Polish Welfare Organisation arranged for a volunteer to take him for weekly car rides. An application was made to the local housing authority for priority rehousing on medical grounds in a ground-floor flat, or a flat in a block with a lift, although it was recognised that rehousing might take several years.

PROGRESS

However, his physical condition steadily deteriorated and six months later it was considered desirable to put his name on the waiting list for a chronic sick bed at his local hospital in case his home care should become impossible. The physician and medical social worker discussed this with Mrs. D and she accepted the suggestion with relief as she was beginning to feel the physical and emotional strain of caring for him. The local welfare authority therefore arranged a two-week holiday for Mr. D at a home especially equipped for severely disabled people. This gave the wife a much needed rest but to Mr. D it further demonstrated his physical dependence on others and his emotional dependence on his wife.

He continued to deteriorate and three months later the physicians considered that further attempts to increase his independence were inappropriate and that he and his wife could best be helped by a programme of planned dependence. The physician therefore suggested to Mr. and Mrs. D in the Outpatient Department that they should both be admitted for a few weeks for assessment and training in home care methods to the Mary Marlborough Lodge, a residential social rehabilitation unit at Oxford for severely disabled people and their relatives. The rehousing claim would be pressed, so that any necessary lifting hoist, grab rails and other gadgets or modifications to the flat could be made before they moved in. Unfortunately, the ambulance driver was in a hurry to take them home from the clinic so it was not realised that they had both misunderstood the doctor's careful explanation and thought that he was recommending Mr. D's permanent admission to a home for disabled people.

The misunderstanding became apparent in a subsequent telephone conversation between Mrs. D and the medical social worker.

Mrs. D was not convinced by the medical social worker's re-explanation and she also denied that the possibility of eventual care in a chronic sick ward had been discussed with her earlier. Before the medical social worker could make a home visit to see both Mr. and Mrs. D in an attempt to clarify the suggested plans, Mr. D made a further suicide attempt and was admitted deeply unconscious to his local hospital.

POINTS TO NOTICE

1. The physician's request for a detailed social investigation and assessment by the medical social worker and a psychiatric opinion.
2. The attempts to improve the patient's mobility and self-care.
3. The concurrent attempts to modify his environment, both physical and emotional, to meet his needs.
4. The ease with which the patient and wife misunderstood the doctor: the difficulty of correcting a misunderstanding once it had arisen and the way in which this influenced the relative's recollection of earlier discussion of care plans.

5. A DISABLED EMPLOYEE

MEDICAL SITUATION

Miss E, aged 45, was a partially-sighted diabetic poorly controlled by diet and insulin. She also had rheumatoid arthritis of the hands.

SOCIAL SITUATION

Miss E was a single woman who had little contact with her relatives who lived in the country. She lived alone in a self-contained flat. She was a very quiet, unassuming woman, a solitary person avoiding the company of others. She was employed as a hand-finisher in the dress workshops of a well-known firm. When her sight deteriorated, she was moved to less exacting work as a dress-machinist but eventually her sight became too bad for her to continue in this employment. During this time the firm continued to employ her and tolerated her hypoglycaemic attacks which increased in frequency as she became more anxious about the future. After a great deal of hesitation she acknowledged that the work was beyond her capabilities and agreed to go to the Industrial Rehabilitation Unit at Egham run by the Department of Employment (formerly the Ministry of Labour) where her abilities could be assessed and a joint decision made as to what kind of work she could undertake.

OCCUPATIONAL RESETTLEMENT

During the six-week assessment period she discovered that there were many types of manual tasks she could manage largely by touch: she also discovered to her surprise that she got on well with her colleagues and staff: she was liked by them and was voted on to the committee of the social club. All this improved her morale very much and she agreed to undertake a six-month training as a dictaphone typist in the Government Training Centre at Egham.

She completed the course satisfactorily and was placed almost at once by the Disablement Resettlement Officer with the Civil Service Commission in a Government department. There she had unbroken employment for five years. As soon as she settled into the job her hypoglycaemic attacks almost ceased. She was apprehensive that the rheumatoid arthritis in her hands might prejudice her new employment but it appeared not to be progressing.

POINTS TO NOTICE

1. The cooperation and understanding of her former employers.
2. The liaison between the hospital physician and medical social worker, the Industrial Rehabilitation Unit, Government Training Centre and Civil Service Commission.
3. The effects of anxiety and then of success and security on her diabetic balance.

6. SOME EFFECTS OF PROGRESSIVE DISABILITY

MEDICAL SITUATION

Mr. F, aged 48, suffered from tabes dorsalis. He had been under medical care continuously for eight years but his physical condition steadily deteriorated and he became chairbound. He retained reasonable strength in his arms and good manual dexterity so that he could operate an indoor wheelchair and an outdoor motor-propelled Invacar (a special car for disabled people provided by the Department of Health).

SOCIAL SITUATION

He was married and his wife worked as an industrial welfare officer but had to give up employment following a nervous breakdown resulting from the strain of her husband's illness. His three children did well at grammar school.

FINANCE AND HOUSING

Owing to Mr. F's long illness and his prolonged periods of unemployment his income dropped from that of a skilled toolmaker to unemployment benefit and he was considerably in debt. He was buying his house on a mortgage but the building society foreclosed on him. Because active resettlement plans were being made, the building society allowed him to remain in the house as their tenant instead of evicting him.

REHABILITATION AND EMPLOYMENT

A medical and social resettlement programme was started which extended over two years. Mr. F went to a medical rehabilitation centre under the National Health Service, where he learned how to use his residual physical ability to the best advantage. He registered as a disabled person under the Disabled Persons'

Employment Act (1944) and the Disablement Resettlement Officer of the Department of Employment placed him as a trainee inspector with a light engineering firm in one of the new towns and found him suitable lodgings there while his family remained in London. Under this scheme of training within industry, the Department of Employment pays a man a training allowance until he begins to be useful to the firm: the employer then pays an increasing proportion of his wages. When he is fully trained, he is taken on the payroll and the Department of Employment's financial contribution to his income ceases. Mr. F completed his training in this way and after one year was taken on the staff.

REHOUSING

When this occurred, he and his family were rehoused in the new town under the Industrial Rehousing Scheme. This is operated jointly by the Department of Employment and the housing departments of the new town corporations. When a man obtains work in a new town through the Department of Employment under this scheme and holds the job satisfactorily for several months, he becomes eligible for rehousing by the corporation.

ATTITUDES

Mr. F had a realistic assessment of the situation and of the effects of his illness on his wife and children. He had a strong sense of responsibility for his family and felt keenly that he had failed them. He was concerned that he might have prejudiced his children's future careers. When he resumed employment, obtained a new house and again became the wage-earner and head of the family, his self-respect improved and he felt less guilty towards his wife and children.

POINTS TO NOTICE

1. The effect of progressive illness on the family relationships and on the family's financial circumstances.

2. The effect of employment on a man's self-respect.
3. The coordinated action, extending over a period of two years, by the patient, the hospital physician and medical social worker, the rehabilitation centre of the National Health Service, the Department of Employment and the new town's housing department.
4. The Department of Employment's training within industry scheme for registered disabled persons.
5. The Industrial Rehousing Scheme.

7. A MARRIED COUPLE WITH MULTIPLE PROBLEMS

MEDICAL SITUATION

Mr. G had suffered from multiple sclerosis for about ten years. He was admitted as a new patient to hospital when his general practitioner discovered that he had developed diabetes mellitus. On admission he needed stabilisation of his diabetes and treatment for extensive pressure sores on his buttocks as he had been confined to bed at home for many months.

SOCIAL SITUATION

Mr. G, aged 49, was married to a wife several years younger: their two children had died in infancy. He was a skilled car mechanic but had been unfit to work for the previous five years and lived on sickness benefit and supplementary allowances. His wife was unable to go out to work as he needed her full-time care. They rented three basement rooms with a kitchen, bedroom and shared lavatory on the ground floor of an old privately-owned house.

Mr. and Mrs. G had strong affection for each other and recognised their mutual emotional dependence but they also had strong feelings of mutual resentment. Mr. G deeply resented and feared his physical dependence on his wife and made himself as helpless as possible in an attempt to tie her more closely to him, and did not recognise that this behaviour was having the opposite effect.

While Mrs. G gained considerable satisfaction at being essential to his welfare, she resented that through his illness she 'had lost her youth' and she looked fifteen years older than her age. She had made a suicide attempt and had several times threatened to leave him unless he cooperated in his care to the best of his ability.

Mr. G was unrealistic in his attitude towards rehabilitation, demanding either complete recovery with return to his former employment or the life of a complete invalid waited on by his wife.

REHABILITATION AND PROGRESS

Mr. G spent eighteen months in hospital. His diabetes was stabilised and he was nursed on a Striker frame for twelve months until his pressure areas had healed. Then his physiotherapy was intensified until he was able to walk with crutches, transfer himself into and out of bed and chair with help and assist with his toilet care and feed himself. Throughout this time he objected to every phase of treatment and was abusive to everyone and especially to his wife.

During the eighteen months the medical social worker tried, with little success, to help Mr. G handle his emotional reactions in a less destructive way and gave additional support to Mrs. G who suffered considerable emotional strain. Their general practitioner, who knew the couple well and regularly visited Mr. G in hospital, suggested that she should get a job. A vacancy was found for her as ward orderly in the hospital on a different ward from her husband's. This enabled her to visit easily and as the domestic staff supervisor and her own ward sister knew of Mr. G, she was treated with considerable understanding.

Concurrently, home care plans were anticipated by the general practitioner, the hospital medical staff, the ward sister, the medical social worker, the physiotherapy and occupational therapy staff. Mr. and Mrs. G were encouraged to take an active part in the planning but he refused to be involved so arrangements were made with Mrs. G.

HOME CARE PLANS

An application was made to the local housing authority for the couple to be rehoused on medical grounds and, as Mr. G was warded for so long, a self-contained ground-floor flat in a modern block was offered before discharge. His mobility and self care were fully assessed in the hospital's Aid to Daily Living Department and the necessary gadgets were determined. The local welfare authority cooperated fully and, before he was discharged, grab-rails were fixed in the lavatory and bathroom, a Warshaw seat was provided in the bath and a ramp was fixed over the one front door step to take the wheel chair provided by the Department of Health.

The district nurse was asked to visit daily for injection of insulin, as Mr. G's tremor prevented him from doing this and Mrs. G was too squeamish to do it for him. He was therefore discharged home to the care of his general practitioner and he attended the out-patient clinic at regular intervals.

HOME CARE DEVELOPMENTS

On reaching home, Mr. G refused to help himself as he had been taught in hospital so Mrs. G had to give up her job to care for him. Relations deteriorated and she made a gesture of leaving him. She then developed a prolapsed intervertebral disc from lifting him and needed outpatient treatment herself. For her home care, a single bed, bedding and fracture board were provided by the local health and welfare authorities and a voluntary organisation. When Mrs. G was physically unable to help him, Mr. G started to help himself. Eventually he developed some pride in his ability to look after himself and to give some little assistance to his wife. Mrs. G made a good recovery and about one year after his discharge they both considered that their relationships were better than they had been for many years. Even when his condition began to deteriorate and he became genuinely more helpless, the home care arrangements remained satisfactory and the relations between Mr. and Mrs. G were those of understanding and cooperation.

POINTS TO NOTICE

1. The success or failure of home care arrangements were entirely dependent on the patient's cooperation.
2. His attitude towards his care was dependent on his attitude towards his wife.
3. The attention paid by the staff to the wife's emotional and then physical needs.
4. The coordinated activity of different departments and personnel.
5. The long-term planning in anticipating needs for home care.
6. The careful medical and social follow-up extending over years.

8. SOME PROBLEMS OF MILD DEMENTIA

MEDICAL SITUATION

Mr. H, aged 67, suffered from mild alcoholic dementia and recurrent malnutrition.

SOCIAL SITUATION

Mr. H lived by himself in two rented rooms on the first floor of a privately-owned house where the lavatory was on the ground floor. His wife was permanently in a mental hospital. Other relatives were a single son and an unmarried sister who took little responsibility for his care and who wanted him admitted compulsorily to a mental hospital. He was physically frail, unsteady on his legs and often somewhat confused and not able to care adequately for himself. But he was too rational for admission to hospital as a formal patient under the Mental Health Act 1959 and he would not accept informal admission to hospital: nor would he agree to enter an old people's home run by the local welfare authority for elderly infirm people.

He therefore remained at home helped by the community care services of the local health and welfare authority. A midday meal was delivered five days a week by the meals-on-wheels service: he had the loan of a commode and he had a home help five days a week to empty the commode and to do cleaning and shopping as required. The district nurse visited once weekly to give him a bath. The arrangements were supervised by the old people's welfare officer of the local welfare authority. The newsagent opposite his home kept a spare key to the house so that the various personnel could let themselves in, and he also called the welfare officer whenever there was a crisis.

However, none of these services operated at the weekends when Mr. H tended to have a drinking bout followed by a week of under-eating. He was therefore periodically brought to hospital in a confused and undernourished state. His physical and mental condition both improved under treatment but as regularly relapsed after he had been home again for several months.

POINTS TO NOTICE

1. The availability of community care services and their co-ordination by a social worker based in the community.
2. The precarious situation of a person too ill to be able to care for himself but not ill enough to justify the representatives of the community taking action to procure his care against his will.

9. PROBLEMS RELATED TO MAJOR SURGERY

Mrs. I, aged 26, suffered from ulcerative colitis and was admitted for colectomy and ileostomy. When Mrs. I declined surgery, the medical social worker was asked to investigate and to help her.

SOCIAL SITUATION

Mrs. I and her husband, a skilled engineering fitter, were Irish Catholics with a son aged two years. Her father had died when she was young and her mother had died two years previously in the same hospital of pyelonephritis. Her only other relative was a single maternal aunt working in Eire.

The family occupied two first-floor rooms in an old privately-owned house. They had a bedroom and living-room, with a gas cooker and sink with a cold water tap on the landing between the rooms. The lavatory was on the ground floor and there was no bath. The lavatory and sink were shared with tenants on the ground floor and both families used the sink for toilet purposes, washing of clothes and preparation of food.

Mrs. I was an immature dependent girl and since her mother's death her aunt had assumed the maternal role. Her ulcerative colitis had started soon after her mother's death and the present exacerbation had started after the aunt's return to Ireland following a holiday in London.

ATTITUDES TO SURGERY

Mrs. I disclosed to the medical social worker that she refused surgery because she was under the impression that a child was born per rectum. She based her belief on the fact that her son had been born shortly after she had had an enema and she concluded that surgical interference with the colon would preclude further pregnancies. Secondly, she was revolted at the thought of an ileostomy and was afraid that her husband would refuse intercourse. The ward sister therefore spent much time teaching her some anatomy and reproductive physiology. Arrangements were then made for her to talk with an older married woman who had successfully managed an ileostomy for several years and lived a full married life. Also, a married male house surgeon discussed these problems with Mrs. I's husband who was then able to give help and encouragement to his wife. Finally, the aunt obtained compassionate leave from her employers and returned to London to care for the child and to give support to Mrs. I. The result was that one week later she consented to surgery and the operation was successfully performed.

PROGRESS

Some six weeks after surgery, Mrs. I went to a Catholic Convent convalescent home where she learned how to manage her ileostomy unaided. On her return home she gradually took over her domestic duties from her aunt who returned to Ireland seven months after the operation. It was considered essential that Mrs. I should move from her present accommodation so that she should have better washing facilities and greater privacy for herself and in order that the public health risk to the two families could be reduced. An application was made to the local housing authority soon after surgery for priority rehousing on medical grounds. After only ten months she was rehoused in a modern self-contained flat consisting of four rooms with separate lavatory and bathroom.

About this time she agreed to join the Ileostomy Association where she met a married woman of her own age who had one child before and another after the fashioning of her ileostomy. Mrs. I's anxieties about her marriage decreased and she and her husband resumed marital relations. She told the medical social worker that she was then living a fuller, happier life than before her operation such as she would not have thought possible a year ago when she was admitted for surgery.

POINTS TO NOTICE

1. The patient's referral to the medical social worker when she refused surgery.
2. Mrs. I's ignorance of anatomy and reproductive physiology and her realistic fears of the effects of an ileostomy on her marriage: both attitudes which had been overlooked by the medical and nursing staff.
3. Her emotional dependence on a mother-figure.
4. The coordinated help given by the medical and nursing staff, the social worker and former patients to both Mrs. I and her husband to help them overcome their emotional difficulties: and the potential value of patient associations such as the Ileostomy Association.

5. The modification of her material environment to meet Mrs. I's needs and in the interests of public health.

10. SOME EFFECTS OF MARITAL DISHARMONY

MEDICAL SITUATION

Mrs. J, aged 46, was referred to the Medical Outpatient Department by her general practitioner complaining of headaches and various pains. She had had a hysterectomy at another hospital four years previously. No organic cause for her headaches was demonstrated and she was diagnosed as suffering from tension pains and depression. The physician referred her to the medical social worker for social investigation and advice.

SOCIAL SITUATION

Mrs. J's parents were dead and her younger married sister lived in the home counties. At the age of 32 she had married a man fifteen years her senior by whom she had a daughter, aged twelve years. Her husband had his own shop selling patent medicines. Before her marriage Mrs. J had held a variety of jobs as shop assistant or typist. After marrying she managed a dress shop for her husband until she had her hysterectomy. Thereafter she managed the accounts for her husband's chemist shop when she felt well enough. Mrs. J gave no details but appeared to be comfortably placed and to be astute over money manners.

Mrs. J, her husband and daughter lived in the flat which Mrs. J had occupied alone as a single woman. It was not self-contained, but the rooms were so placed that no other tenants came through her part of the house. The accommodation consisted of one living-room, one bedroom, small kitchen, lavatory and bathroom. In the bedroom, Mrs. J and her daughter shared a double bed and her husband had a single bed.

It became clear on taking the social history that, following the birth of her daughter, Mr. and Mrs. J had moved slowly apart, she occupying herself with the child to the exclusion of her husband

and he concentrating on his business and many masonic activities which excluded her. Marital relations ceased early in the marriage and they had had the present sleeping arrangements for many years. They lived separate lives alongside each other, had no shared interests in the home or family and discussed nothing of importance together.

Mrs. J was extremely sensitive to other people's opinions. She said that she had been ashamed to admit to the doctor in what 'squalor' she lived and she and her daughter had few friends as, for the same reason, they did not invite them home. She despised her neighbours, emphasised how the district had 'gone down' over the years and wanted to move somewhere 'classy'. She sent her daughter to a fee-paying school. She presented all this as being more hurtful to her self-esteem than the failure of her marriage and she attributed her illness to the emotional stress of her material environment. She thought that her husband was quite content with the present arrangements and would not consider additional expenditure on accommodation as he was nearing retirement.

ACTION

As the marital difficulties were of such long standing and as Mrs. J did not acknowledge that they were of prime importance in her illness, the medical social worker considered that it was more appropriate to approach the marital problem through the housing problem rather than directly. It was possible that the harmful effect of overcrowding on the child would provide an area in which Mr. and Mrs. J might start to act jointly and thereby improve their relationship. The medical social worker therefore redefined the problem to her in these terms. Over the next four months she saw Mrs. J at fortnightly intervals and the physician saw her monthly. The medical social worker gave advice on effecting exchange of tenancies and advertising and also gave practical help with letters to her landlord's agent. At each stage she encouraged Mrs. J to discuss each proposed action with her husband and obtain his consent. Mr. and Mrs. J slowly re-established some degree of cooperation and a sense of joint responsibility so that Mr. J no longer left her to take all the initiative in looking for more suitable accommodation. Concurrently Mrs. J's pains and depression decreased. Eventually she decided that she and her husband could continue to look for accommodation without the social worker's help. Shortly after, the physician referred her back to her general practitioner with the offer that she could return to see him or the medical social worker whenever she felt it necessary.

POINTS TO NOTICE

1. The careful assessment of the relative importance of different aetiological factors.
2. The patient's attitude towards the material and emotional factors, the former being 'acceptable', the latter not.
3. The social worker's use of the few strong points in the situation, namely the parents' concern for their daughter's well-being, Mrs. J's business acumen, her strong motivation to move house.
4. The policy of supporting the patient until she felt able to cope unaided.

11. AN UNMARRIED MOTHER'S BABY

BABY AND MOTHER

Kenneth was admitted to the Infectious Disease Unit suffering from a Salmonella infection only three weeks after he had left the Maternity Unit with his mother.

She was an unmarried West Indian and the putative father of Kenneth, her first child, disclaimed paternity. The mother occupied a poorly appointed, rented bed-sitting-room and shared the lavatory and washing facilities with other tenants. She was not working so soon after delivery and was receiving statutory allowances from the Department of Social Security.

MOTHER'S ATTITUDE

The mother could not accept her rejection by the putative father and attempted to use the baby as a means of reinstating herself in a liaison with him. He was not prepared to be manipulated in this way and already had another girl friend. The mother, in common with many women, did not wish to make a legal application through the Magistrate's Court for a maintenance allowance for the child.

Her attitude to her baby was as ambivalent as that towards the putative father. She was therefore unable to make realistic plans for the baby's future and to decide whether to try to maintain him herself or to relinquish him to adopters. The baby's admission to hospital enabled her to postpone the unpleasantness of decision and by visiting the baby daily in hospital she was able to reassure herself that she was fulfilling her maternal role.

FUTURE PLANNING

The baby's hospital stay was prolonged as it was impossible to discharge him until he was free of infection. At intervals, members of the hospital staff, including the ward sister and medical social worker, saw the mother and encouraged her to think about the future. During these conversations, her own history came to light. Following a common cultural pattern in the West Indies, her parents were not married but neither were they living in a stable union in a common law marriage. Her own mother left her as a child in the care of the maternal grandmother while she came to England. She trained and worked as a nurse and subsequently married. The daughter then came to England herself to work. She met her mother but felt herself to be an embarrassment and their relationship was very strained. So far, Kenneth's mother was following the same pattern of life as her own mother.

It was difficult for the hospital staff to accept the young mother's emotional immaturity and instability and to recognise that she must be allowed to come to her own decision about her role as a mother: and that before she could do this, she needed to express the extremes of her uncertainties and hostility about the baby, the putative father and the hospital staff. It was recognised that if she were to be pushed into making a particular decision she might well reverse it later and cause distress as well as waste of time. In moods of depression she talked of suicide. The psychiatrist who saw her considered that she was not suffering from a puerperal depression but was reacting to her social difficulties and feelings of rejection.

Seven months after admission, Kenneth was free from infection and the mother was told she would shortly have to make a decision on his future. The medical social worker put her in touch with the local child care officer to discuss the possibility of placing Kenneth in a residential nursery or foster home under the care of the local children's department, if she wished to keep him and resume work to support him. She was also told how to make arrangements for his adoption if she wanted this. Eventually, she effected a compromise which was both realistic and acceptable to her. She applied to the child care officer for the baby to be placed in a residential nursery, where she could contribute towards his maintenance and visit him regularly while, again like her mother, she proposed to train as a nurse.

POINTS TO NOTICE

1. The mother's ambivalent feelings towards the baby and her consequent inability to decide on his and her future. (This difficulty may have been accentuated by cultural differences between Barbados and England.)
2. The understanding by the hospital staff of her emotional difficulties and their tolerance of her hostility.
3. The similarity between the mother's experiences and those of her own mother.

12. SOME PROBLEMS OF OLD AGE

MEDICAL SITUATION

Mrs. L was aged 87 and suffered from rectal incontinence. She was mentally alert but very deaf.

SOCIAL SITUATION

Mrs. L was a widow, maintaining herself on her old age pension and supplementary allowance. She occupied one room in the house which for many years had been her family home. The lavatory and water supply were on a different floor and she found the stairs increasingly difficult to negotiate. The remainder of the house was occupied by her only close relatives, her married son and his wife, both of whom were out at work during the day.

DOMICILIARY CARE

Mrs. L received a cooked meal delivered daily by the meals-on-wheels service and a home help came for a few hours each week to do the cleaning and shopping. A visitor from a local voluntary social work organisation called periodically to maintain contact. Her son and his wife called in daily on their return from work but their visits were perfunctory and they gave no help and little companionship. The domestic needs were therefore met but the problem remained one of loneliness and isolation with no help available in emergencies.

HOSPITAL ADMISSION AND DISCHARGE PLANS

After Mrs. L had suffered an acute exacerbation of rectal incontinence, her general practitioner decided that she was unfit for treatment at home and her admission to hospital was arranged. After treatment her condition improved and discharge and after-care plans were considered.

LOOKING AT THE PROBLEM WITH THE PATIENT

When the medical social worker was informed of the patient's medical situation, she arranged a private interview with Mrs. L away from the ward in view of her deafness and the nature of the problem to be discussed. The social worker introduced herself and carefully explained the purpose of the interview. Mrs. L recognised the concern for her welfare and readily discussed her difficulties. She valued her relationship with her son and daughter-in-law: she appreciated their difficulties and was not bitter at their partial rejection of her. She therefore asked to be admitted to an old people's home.

LOOKING AT THE PROBLEM WITH THE RELATIVES

During Mrs. L's admission the relatives visited regularly but asked the ward staff only about her condition and avoided discussion of discharge plans. The social worker asked them to visit her to discuss after-care plans and, although the latter did not define any attitude or plans, they arrived bristling with hostility. The social worker asked them to describe the situation as they saw it. They described the difficulties of the past year, referring to gas taps being left on, the risks of burning and scalding, Mrs. L's personal uncleanliness and occasions of collapse, and stated their unwillingness and inability to resume any responsibility. When they did not receive the criticism that they were expecting, they gradually relaxed and were able to reassess the practical and emotional difficulties of caring for an elderly frail person. The practical issues were discussed first: the possibility of rearranging the use of rooms to facilitate use of lavatory and taps: the local authority special laundry service for incontinent patients. The relatives left to consider suggestions, with their own difficulties recognised but with their role as important participators in the planning mutually acknowledged.

OLD PEOPLE'S HOME

It was eventually agreed between the patient, her relatives and the hospital staff, that Mrs. L would apply for admission to a home run by the local welfare authority (so-called Part III accommodation). The local authority welfare officer came to see her in hospital to assess her suitability for their homes. Some were small purpose-built homes but others were large institutional-type buildings and there was a long waiting-list for all. Mrs. L was able to be up and to dress herself with a little help but her mobility was poor and she was still incontinent at night. Therefore the local authority considered her unfit for admission.

GERIATRIC HOSPITAL

Mrs. L was therefore referred to the geriatrician in charge of the long-stay beds for Mrs. L's home area: the physician's letter gave medical particulars and enclosed a social report from the social worker. Her name was put on the waiting-list, which was very long.

PRIVATE HOME

Mrs. L was a border-line case, her medical condition falling between the criteria set for admission to a welfare authority home and to a geriatric long-stay ward. Homes run by voluntary organisations are often suitable for such patients as the regulations are more flexible and the staff have more freedom of choice over admissions. One particular organisation was building a new wing to one of its homes which would be suitable for Mrs. L. The organisation's welfare officer visited Mrs. L in the ward and arranged with her to put her name on the list for admission as soon as the wing was opened.

POINTS TO NOTICE

1. The patient's insight into her problems and those of her relatives.
2. The way in which the patient was encouraged to participate actively in planning her own future.
3. The way in which the cooperation of the relatives was enlisted in constructive planning and their own difficulties in the situation were recognised without any recrimination.
4. The permissive attitude of the hospital staff. If an authoritarian attitude had been adopted and the patient sent home

under circumstances which her general practitioner considered to be inadequate and against the wishes of the patient and her relatives, it was probable that readmission would have been necessary. In addition, the confidence of the patient and the cooperation of the relatives would have been forfeited by the hospital staff and the relationship between Mrs. L and her relatives would have deteriorated further, causing more unhappiness.

5. If Mrs. L had insisted on returning home against the wishes of her relatives, the hospital staff and her general practitioner would have had to cooperate with her, as such a decision must rest with the patient. Many old people will tolerate the discomforts and risks entailed in living at home for the sake of their familiar surroundings and to escape from the dependence and impersonalisation which some of them feel under any kind of institutional care.

13. A PROBLEM OF PERSONAL RELATIONSHIPS

MEDICAL SITUATION

Mrs. M, aged 30, attended her general practitioner complaining of abdominal pain. He examined her but could find no cause for her symptoms which were suggestive of early peptic ulceration. He advised her on diet and prescribed an antacid. She attended again three weeks later complaining of headache. Once again no abnormality was detected. At her third consultation within a period of two months her complaint was of pruritus vulvae. Physical examination was again negative. The doctor asked her to return for another appointment when he could allow her the time for a lengthy interview.

SOCIAL HISTORY

Mrs. M was born and bred in London. She came from a stable working class home and had one brother and one sister. Her health in childhood was good but she suffered from hay fever in her teens. She related well to her parents, siblings and to children at school. When she left school at the age of 15 she obtained steady employment in a food store.

She had a number of boy friends before she met her husband at the age of 19. She went out with him for two years and during the second year enjoyed sexual intercourse with him. She felt that this was wrong and that her mother would have disapproved had she known. She was therefore very distressed to find herself pregnant before marriage. She tried a number of remedies reputed to be of value but none produced the desired abortion. Her fiancé married her and in due course she gave birth to a son, Alan. She was horrified to discover that he was born with a hare lip and cleft palate. Two years later she was delivered of a normal boy, Robert.

Mr. M came from a stable home and was a hard-working painter and decorator. He provided well for his family who had no financial problems and lived in a comfortable council flat. He rarely attended the doctor but when he came he was not very communicative.

Alan was treated in early life by plastic surgery. Now, aged ten, he had made good progress at school and his only troublesome illness was flexural eczema. Robert was a normal healthy boy, aged eight.

IMMEDIATE PROBLEMS

Mrs. M presented two problems in her long interview with the doctor. The first was the fact that she had not enjoyed sexual intercourse with her husband since marriage. She said she was unable to discuss this with him and indeed found it difficult to communicate with him at all. Her second problem was due to the fact that Alan had to return to the plastic surgeon at the age of eleven for readmission to hospital for further surgery. She had not told him about this and did not know how to broach the subject with him. She spent sleepless nights worrying about this but she could not discuss it with her husband.

PROGRESS

The general practitioner arranged a joint interview with Mr. and Mrs. M in which he acted as interpreter between them and helped them to discuss their sexual relationship. This opened up a new avenue of communication in their marriage. The general practitioner also advised them how to tell Alan of his impending re-admission to hospital. When he was told, his reaction was, 'Oh, good! When do I go in?"

Following these interviews Mrs. M became symptom free.

POINTS TO NOTICE

1. Mrs. M presented her general practitioner with symptoms of physical illness. He could not explain these until he elicited her underlying anxiety and the causes for it.
2. Mrs. M reacted in a predictable way to her pre-marital pregnancy: but the birth of a deformed child filled her with guilt about her initial rejection of him by her attempts to procure an abortion and she felt responsible for his deformity.
3. These guilt feelings were probably responsible for her subsequent attitude to sexual intercourse.
4. The inability of Mr. and Mrs. M to discuss these intimate problems made the situation more difficult for her.
5. The prospect of telling her son of the need for further treatment for the deformity for which she felt responsible increased her anxiety to an intolerable level. She then developed physical symptoms for which she sought medical advice.
6. The treatment provided by the general practitioner consisted of help to improve the personal relationships between Mrs. M and her husband and son.

14. THE DISRUPTIVE EFFECTS OF SERIOUS ILLNESS

MEDICAL HISTORY

Mr. N, aged 72, developed a chest infection which his general practitioner treated with antibiotics. Although he responded well to treatment the abnormal physical signs in his chest persisted. A chest X-ray revealed a carcinoma of the bronchus. He was a heavy smoker.

SOCIAL HISTORY

Mr. N was born in London and lived in the suburbs throughout his working life. At the age of 24 he married a woman four years older than himself. He was a successful small tradesman and only retired at the age of 70. On his retirement they moved to a bungalow in the West Country but could not tolerate the peace and quiet of the countryside, became lonely and returned to London six months before the onset of his illness. They occupied the ground floor of their house and were comfortably provided for materially.

The younger of their two sons (both now in their forties) occupied the first floor of their house and was employed in the television industry. The elder son had made a disastrous marriage and had run into debt from which his father extricated him, but there was little contact between them now.

Mr. N had always enjoyed very good health and led an active life until the onset of his illness. He had a strong personality and appeared to make most of the decisions for the family. His wife's health had been less good in recent years and this had increased her already considerable dependence on him.

PROGRESS

Mr. N recovered from his acute illness unaware of the underlying carcinoma. He was, however, far less active than before and found it difficult to get out of the house. He very much resented his invalidism.

Mrs. N was deeply distressed on being told of her husband's diagnosis and reacted aggressively to the failure of the medical profession to cure her husband.

Over the next few months Mr. N's condition steadily

deteriorated. In particular he became very depressed, had difficulty in concentrating and his memory became impaired. His wife was very intolerant of his shortcomings and on one occasion when he wet the bed she reacted as if to a medical emergency and felt unable to continue with his care at home.

The general practitioner therefore arranged for a domiciliary consultation with a physician when it was decided to admit him to hospital. He improved almost immediately, began to get about more and to take a renewed interest in life. After two weeks he was discharged home. Within a week he had taken to his bed and become deeply depressed.

ATTITUDES TO ILLNESS

At this stage Mr. N's attitude was one of depression and despondency about himself. Mrs. N had a deep resentment of her husband's increasing invalidism and of his dependence on her. She had an intense fear of cancer which increased her anxiety. The son provided no support in this situation and strenuously recommended admission to hospital.

TERMINAL CARE

The general practitioner tried to take the pressure off Mrs. N by arranging for a home help to undertake some of the domestic work. A district nurse was asked to visit daily. Her nursing role was minimal but she did a great deal to restore the morale of the family.

After several weeks Mr. N fell in his bedroom and was not discovered for some hours by his wife. The general practitioner arranged his admission to hospital where he died two weeks later.

POINTS TO NOTICE

1. The onset of serious physical illness in an aggressively independent man led to severe depression.
2. His over-dependent wife resented his increasing invalidism

and his dependence on her caused her extreme anxiety. Her overwhelming fear of cancer exacerbated the situation. No relief was provided by inadequate sons.

3. Close cooperation and sympathetic understanding by a district nurse and home help improved the situation temporarily but it was not possible for the patient to die peacefully at home.
4. The reaction of both the patient and his wife to his illness might have been different if he had been told what was the matter with him and he had been able to discuss it with his wife.

PART III

THE MEDICAL AND SOCIAL SERVICES

INTRODUCTION

MEMBERS OF THE TEAM

The practice of clinical medicine involves a body of knowledge and the application of techniques drawn from a number of different disciplines. These fall into two main groups, namely the established biological and physical sciences and the developing behavioural sciences. The practice of scientific medicine involves the use of scientific method in diagnosis, treatment and clinical research, together with the application of advanced techniques largely developed by the physical sciences. The fundamental procedure in scientific method is the formulation and testing of an hypothesis under controlled conditions in which the effect of the observer is reduced to a minimum. Thus in diagnosis the clinician formulates his hypothesis or provisional diagnosis from data obtained from the history and physical examination. To test the hypothesis a variety of investigations may be necessary involving the use of techniques derived from other disciplines. Similarly he may use methods of treatment, and methods of assessing the effectiveness of treatment, derived from a variety of disciplines. These may be physiology, biochemistry, pharmacology, physics and mathematics on the one hand, and psychology, sociology and social anthropology on the other. In this latter group, the aspects that particularly concern the clinician are elements of normal developmental psychology with some knowledge of dynamic psychology and of the meaning of illness to the individual: elements of social psychology especially factors affecting social perception and group behaviour: some knowledge of cultural patterns of behaviour and in particular those governing behaviour during illness and response to illness in others.

As the clinician cannot be an expert in all these fields, he enlists the assistance of a number of medical and non-medical professional personnel to provide the required detailed knowledge and skills. Thus the practice of clinical medicine increasingly involves the exercise of a variety of skills by members of a team, whose leader and coordinator is the clinician who has the ultimate responsibility for the patient.

Developments of medical practice over the last hundred years have resulted in a two tier structure in clinical practice. The general practitioner, or family doctor, is the professional man in direct contact with the lay public who are his patients. He has now acquired the additional role of leader of the professional team that practises in the community. The hospital specialist or consultant has no such direct contact with the public and receives his patients by referral from the family doctor, to whose care the patients return after the consultation or on completion of specialised treatment. The consultant practises in hospital (and often also in his private consulting rooms) and is the leader of the hospital-based team. Since most general hospitals are now 'district' hospitals with a recognised duty to provide service for a defined population, the hospital staff are becoming increasingly aware of community needs and the problems of home care.

THE COMMUNITY TEAM

MEDICAL PERSONNEL

THE FAMILY DOCTOR

Not only is the family doctor or general practitioner the leader of the community team but in a real sense he is at the centre of the patient's care. It has been said that 'only general practice can ensure that the patient is treated both as an individual and in relation to his family background, and it alone provides for continuity of treatment at all times by one doctor' and 'the general practitioner, by the exercise of his responsibility for the patient, can link together preventive, social and curative medicine'. (Central Health Services Council, *Report of the Committee on General Practice within the Health Service*, 1954, H.M.S.O., pp. 2–3.)

There are approximately 20,400 family doctors in practice in the National Health Service. Each of these doctors has a 'list' of patients for whom he is paid on a per capita basis whether or not the patients require medical treatment. The average list is 2500 patients for a single-handed practice but the number varies with the geographical area, the density of population, the number of local practices and the preference of the doctor. Increasingly general practitioners are working in group practices of four, five or six doctors. This enables specialisation within the practice and administratively it facilitates off-duty and night-call rotas and the employment or 'attachment' of non-medical personnel and of secretarial help. When the Health Service was instituted in 1948, the establishment of health centres was to be a central feature of general practice but this concept is only now gaining acceptance.

A health centre is usually owned by the local health authority (see page 126). It consists of a series of consulting rooms and offices and is equipped with diagnostic and treatment facilities. Accommodation and use of the facilities is then rented by local group practices. As this policy becomes more widespread, it is expected that general practitioners will cease to run their surgeries in their own houses and that eventually the health centre will also have medical and non-medical members of the local health and welfare authorities working in the community alongside the family doctor (see following pages).

INFANT WELFARE CLINIC DOCTOR

The local health authority (see page 126) provides a well-baby clinic in each administrative area for the supervision of infants at regular intervals from the age of about fourteen days to five years. The physician in charge may be a full-time employee of the health authority or a local family doctor employed on a sessional basis. His role is to screen the babies for evidence of congenital or early acquired disease and to watch their physical and mental development. He refers them, if necessary, to their family doctors for treatment or for decisions about specialist consultation.

SCHOOL MEDICAL OFFICER

The local education authority (see page 126) provides a medical service in its schools to screen children on entering school at five years of age, often again at eleven years and before leaving at fifteen. School medical officers responsible for administration of the service are usually full-time local authority employees but those running the school clinics are often general practitioners or married women doctors employed on a sessional basis. Any treatment required is arranged in consultation with the child's family doctor. It may be carried out by the school medical service, by the general practitioner or by referral to hospital for specialist care.

MEDICAL OFFICER OF HEALTH

The Principal Medical Officer of a local health authority is normally also the Principal School Medical Officer. His full-time assistants may also have a similar dual role but more often each has special responsibility for some aspect of the school medical service or of the local health authority's functions in the field of public health or the provision of personal care services (see page 126). These services are supplied at the request of or in co-operation with the family doctor.

STUDENT HEALTH SERVICE

Such a service is operated by a university to provide a general practitioner service to students during term if they are away from home. This is both a preventive and therapeutic service and treatment is given in conjunction with the family doctor.

INDUSTRIAL HEALTH SERVICE

The local education authority (see page 126) provides a medical ments for good working conditions and provisions for first aid in case of accident or injury. Appointed Factory Doctors, often local general practitioners, are appointed by the Department of Employment and Productivity to examine young persons and selected groups of workers, and to report on cases of notifiable industrial disease and accidents resulting in injury or death.

Many large industrial organisations provide a well-developed industrial health service with full-time medical and nursing personnel. In addition to meeting the statutory requirements described above, such a service can provide continuing advice to management on medical aspects of industrial processes, advise on the rehabilitation of injured or sick employees, provide emergency treatment in cases of an accident and ongoing treatment in conjunction with the employee's general practitioner.

The Tunbridge Report (1968) made recommendations for such an occupational health service for employees in National Health Service hospitals.

NURSING PERSONNEL

THE DISTRICT NURSE

The district nurse is a State Registered Nurse with additional training in the specialised demands of domiciliary nursing and her function is to nurse people in their own homes. The system was started in 1859 by William Rathbone, a merchant in Liverpool, who realised that poor people were not benefiting fully from medical treatment owing to inadequate nursing. Voluntary district nursing associations were founded all over the country, and the Queen's Institute for District Nursing was formed to coordinate their work and standards and to provide training courses. With the introduction of the Health Service, home nursing became the responsibility of the local health authorities who, to a large extent, have maintained the service by subsidising existing district nursing associations.

Each district nurse, or home nurse as she is often called, has her own district and provides the nursing care requested by general practitioners or hospital doctors. She usually visits a home once or twice a day to assist with bed-making and bathing, to give injections, do dressings and to administer those drugs that are covered by the Dangerous Drugs Act and cannot be administered by unqualified people. Usually she supplies the skilled component of nursing care to supplement the unskilled care given by relatives and friends. However, she will train a patient or relative how to perform a semi-skilled procedure, such as giving a diabetic an injection of insulin, and supervise his or her progress until she is satisfied that it is being competently performed.

Under the Health Service, the district nursing associations only provide care during the day. However, in some areas the nursing associations have arrangements with a voluntary organisation, the Marie Curie Foundation, whereby the association provides a night nursing service which the Foundation supports financially, for patients with cancer who require skilled attention at night.

The devoted care given by district nurses enables many chronically sick or elderly people and those in the terminal stages of illness to remain at home with their families or in their own familiar surroundings instead of being admitted to hospital. Not only does this provide help and comfort to the patient and his family but it also frees more hospital beds for those patients for whom full-time skilled nursing care is essential.

THE MIDWIFE

Midwives always have a training in midwifery and are usually State Registered Nurses. Since 1902, when the Central Midwives' Board was founded, this body has supervised training and examined pupil midwives and, as no midwife can practise unless she is a certificated and registered midwife, has ensured high standards of professional competence. Since 1936 the local health authority has been responsible for providing a domiciliary midwifery service. They usually do this by employing the midwives themselves but in some areas the local authority subsidises a voluntary organisation, such as the District Nursing Association, to provide the personnel and the service.

Approximately half the deliveries (49·8 per cent) in Great Britain are performed by a midwife, and in nearly half (48·5 per cent) she is the senior person present. Approximately 36 per cent are performed in the patient's home. (Butler and Bonham 1963.)

THE HEALTH VISITOR

The health visitor is a State Registered Nurse who has completed at least part one of the midwifery training and has had further training in public health and preventive medicine. The Working Party on Health Visitors has described her function as 'primarily that of health education and social advice'. In considering the complementary functions of a health visitor and social worker, the Report of the Ministry of Health Working Party on Social Workers in Local Authority Health and Welfare Services (Younghusband Committee 1959) stated: 'The value and importance of the work of health visitors is well recognised, notably in improving the health of mothers and young children and raising the standards of child care, and in the follow-up of the sick and chronic sick discharged from hospital, in promoting the health of the elderly, in the care of the tuberculous and whenever special diets are required or other aspects of medical treatment must be considered. Their work in these spheres inevitably brings them into contact with a variety of social problems. It is desirable that their training should enable them, in the course of their normal duties, to recognise the signs of these and that they should have a good understanding of the functions of other workers, so as to refer cases appropriately. . . . The great asset of the health visitor in the social sphere is her knowledge of the treatment and prevention of disease and the promotion of health.' (Part IV. Chapter 10, paras 961 and 962.)

The health visitor is an employee of the local health authority and is usually based in an infant welfare centre run by that authority but may be seconded to work with groups of general practitioners. On receipt of a notification of birth from the Medical Officer of Health she has a statutory duty to visit the mother and child in their home. She has no right of entry but relies on the public's acceptance of health visitors and her own tact to establish a good professional relationship with the mother. This enables her to offer any help needed on feeding or management difficulties and to arrange for the mother to bring the infant to see the clinic doctor. She continues to visit the family at intervals according to their need and arranges the periodic medical examination of the infant until he reaches the age of five years. Mothers often consult her on a wide range of medical and social problems, and when necessary she refers them to the appropriate doctor, social worker or other source of help.

Health visitor attachments to general practice are increasing especially where group practices are developing. By arrangement with the local health authority, a health visitor whose area most closely corresponds with that of a practice is allocated to work with the doctor. The method of cooperation varies: some doctors telephone their health visitors only when they have cases to refer:

many have regular meetings for referral of new cases and discussions of progress in current cases. In other practices, the health visitors attend the surgeries, in particular the baby clinics run by practitioners with a domiciliary obstetric practice. In some areas such general practitioners hold their baby clinics in the premises of the infant welfare centre, so that close cooperation with health visitors over infant care is possible even if there is no formal health visitor attachment. When infants are supervised by the general practitioner in this way, they seldom attend the local authority infant welfare clinic as well.

The cases referred to health visitors by general practitioners, medical social workers and others are usually those involving some medical aspect of infant or child care and follow-up of sick, chronic sick or elderly people at home.

THE SCHOOL NURSE

The school nurse is a member of the school medical service of the local education authority. She attends the school clinics with the school medical officer: in some areas she arranges the medical examinations and follows up recommendations and referrals for treatment to ensure that they are carried out, either by the school medical service, the general practitioner or by referral to hospital for specialist treatment.

As the school nurse for any particular school is often the health visitor for the district, she often knows the children from the days when they attended the infant welfare centre or she currently knows their pre-school-age brothers and sisters. She is thus able to give the school medical officer valuable information about the child's home and upbringing so that he can be considered, not as an isolated individual, but as a member of a family. By this means the health visitor in her dual role is able to be a family health visitor, a development recommended in the report of the Chief Medical Officer of the then Ministry of Education in 1961. In this way her task of obtaining the active cooperation of the child's parents in his treatment is facilitated. Her role as health educator makes her a suitable person to take classes in personal hygiene, the physiology of reproduction and sex education for the older children, particularly as many health visitors are married with children of their own.

In some areas of London her tasks of liaison with the child's home, with general practitioners and hospitals are carried out by a voluntary worker from the school's care committee (see page 103) while in other parts of the country the nurse's less skilled duties are performed by lay assistants.

SOCIAL WORKERS

Another group of non-medical personnel with whom doctors may cooperate are social workers. There is nowadays a bewildering variety of trained and untrained social workers based in the community to serve different groups of people, having different functions and with different training or experience. This situation arose because most of the existing social services developed over the last 150 years as voluntary services more or less in isolation. Then a number were taken over by the central or local government as statutory services once the need for them was proved. All these services 'minister in some way to the personal wellbeing of individual members of the community, but they differ in scope, purpose, approach and method of administration. Moreover, in the main, their growth has been haphazard, since they came into being one by one as the community, or at any rate the more sensitive among its members, became aware of personal needs to be met or social evils to be overcome.' (Hall 1963, p. 344.)

An attempt is now being made to bring some order into the situation by considering first the different types of social difficulties that people may experience, and then by considering the different types of training that social workers may require in order to help people with these difficulties. A great step forward was taken with the publication of the Younghusband Report in 1959. By its terms of reference the report was limited to considering the local authority services only but many of its recommendations are being implemented in other social services.

The report considered that the needs of people for social work help fall into three broad categories. While it is obvious that people's difficulties do not fall neatly into categories, as an individual may experience several difficulties simultaneously, this three-fold classification is a useful guide when considering the function of a social service and the calibre and training of the social workers required to staff it.

First is the need for simple explanation about existing relevant services, about pension rights and other factual information. This may be of crucial importance to the individual but from the social worker it requires primarily sympathy, understanding and a body of factual knowledge. It was considered that a person of suitable temperament could satisfactorily undertake this work after a short period of in-service training; such a person would be known as a welfare assistant.

The second category consists of fairly obvious and straightforward, although more severe difficulties, such as the need for rehousing, for domestic help, for home nursing, for the relief of loneliness. Here the social worker must first establish a relationship with the person, investigate the social situation by collecting relevant information, make a social 'diagnosis', discuss with the individual the best ways of meeting his needs, and help him or her to implement the agreed course of action, the equivalent of 'treatment'. It was recommended that such 'general purpose' caseworkers should have a two year full-time training and special courses leading to a certificate in general social work have been established in many colleges of further education. These courses usually include the study of social history, economics, human growth and development, social administration and the theory and practice of casework, with periods of supervised practical field work. Many untrained social workers are being seconded by their employing local authorities to take this training and also older men and women with relevant previous experience are now entering social work in this way.

Finally, there are the social problems of considerable complexity especially those which arise through disturbances in personal relationships and through personality disorders. It was considered that these people could best be helped by professionally trained caseworkers. These social workers take a three year university degree course in social science covering sociology, psychology, social history and social administration. Students who have already graduated in another faculty may take a one year post-graduate diploma briefly covering the same subjects, while for older non-graduates with an adequate educational background there is a special two year university diploma course in social science. Each of these basic university courses is then followed by a one year professional training in the theory and practice of casework. So that a professionally trained caseworker has followed a course of university and professional training lasting three, four or five years.

It has already been shown that the practice of casework involves four stages, namely the establishment of a professional relationship: social investigation: social 'diagnosis': and 'treatment' which is agreed upon by the client and those concerned and implemented jointly by social worker and client. The professional relationship is 'one which will support and strengthen the client and enable him to make better use of the community services available to him. In the establishment and maintenance of this relationship the outlook and attitudes of the worker are all-important.' (Hall, 1963, p. 133.) Here, the influence of dynamic psychology is evident and during the last fifty years the emphasis in social work 'has shifted from social conditions and circumstances as they affect the client and how they can be put right, not least by his own efforts, to personal relationships and how they can be adjusted. Nevertheless, economic realities cannot be ignored, and environmental influences, including the traditions and mores of the particular group or culture to which the client belongs, are both influential and important. Thus the social worker must take into account economic and social as well as psychological factors in diagnosing a situation, and incorporate the knowledge gained from economics, sociology and social research into her thinking along with that gained from psychiatry and psychology.' (ibid., p. 135.) Another consequence of the psychological approach is that the modern social worker is less moralistic in her attitude than her predecessors and 'is more likely to try to discover and understand the reasons for her client's behaviour than to assess his or her moral responsibility. . . . Along with this approach goes a strong reluctance to impose one's own standards on those with different traditions and social norms.' (ibid., p. 135.)

Casework was first practised at the end of the last century by social workers in a voluntary organisation now known as the Family Welfare Association. In 1895 one of these caseworkers was appointed to the Royal Free Hospital in London and thus became the first almoner and the first caseworker to apply her skills in a specialised setting where the main function was to provide not social work help but medical care. The almoners (now known as medical social workers) increased in number and were later joined by other caseworkers with a slightly different role, the psychiatric social workers. In the field of jurisprudence, other caseworkers succeeded the former officers of the Police Court Mission and the Probation Service came into being under the aegis of the Home Office. Later still, other caseworkers were appointed under the Home Office to start the Child Care Service of the local authority.

The methods of casework used in all these settings are the same but are applied to meet the needs of particular groups of people. However, the professional training courses in casework are usually a specialised preparation for work in one particular field, as each course was developed separately to equip social workers to practise in one particular setting. As part of the process of rationalising social work practice and training, several universities now run a 'generic' or 'applied' course in casework for students who have completed the basic academic training. These applied courses are accepted by the appropriate professional organisations and employing authorities as qualifying the social worker to practise casework in several fields. This common training not only improves communication between caseworkers in different fields but enables the individual social worker to move from one setting to another without the necessity of obtaining a further professional qualification first.

Although both men and women become social workers, the

proportion of men varies in the different types of work, being low in medical social work and family casework and rather higher in psychiatric social work, child care and probation.

MEDICAL AND PSYCHIATRIC SOCIAL WORKERS

The first medical social worker at the Royal Free Hospital had two main duties: first, to ensure that those people who could afford to pay for treatment were not treated free as a charity by a voluntary hospital and, secondly, to help those patients who had social difficulties which were causing illness or delaying recovery. Since the introduction of the Health Service in 1948 the medical social worker has been relieved of the first duty which involved a 'means test'. Now she works in close cooperation with doctors to supplement medical care. She may assist in diagnosis by uncovering social factors relevant to the aetiology of the patient's disease. She may cooperate in treatment by helping the patient suitably to modify his environment or to adjust to a different way of life necessitated by a chronic disease or disability. Although the patient is the focus of her attention, he cannot be considered in isolation and in some cases much of her time is spent helping his immediate relatives so that he may ultimately benefit from their greater understanding and cooperation. The medical social worker helps patients who have predominantly physical illness or disability. The psychiatric social worker fulfils a similar function with patients whose illness or handicap is primarily psychological. However, there is no hard boundary as many people with a physical illness have emotional difficulties related to it while the mentally ill or handicapped may also suffer from physical disease.

The medical social worker has taken a basic university degree or diploma course in social science followed by a professional casework course, either an applied course, a specialised course run by the Institute of Medical Social Workers, or a university course in medical social work approved by the Institute. There are approximately 1200 trained medical social workers in Great Britain.

The psychiatric social worker has also taken a basic university degree or diploma course in social science followed by a professional casework course, either an applied course or a university course in psychiatric social work approved by the Association of Psychiatric Social Workers. There are approximately 900 trained psychiatric social workers in Great Britain.

Medical and psychiatric social workers who are based in the community are usually employed in the local authority's health and welfare services (see page 126). Although as yet very few are employed in this way the number is increasing as the medical care of the physically or mentally ill or handicapped is shifting from hospitals into the community. They usually occupy the senior or advisory posts as recommended by the Younghusband Report and are part of a team of social workers including general social workers and in-service trained welfare assistants. In these terms, the different members carry the cases which they are best equipped to help. Because of the rapid expansion of the local authority health and welfare services during the last twenty years and the shortage of trained social workers, there are many untrained social workers in these services. Some have obtained a basic social science qualification but no social work qualification, while others have had no formal training. Nevertheless, many of the older social workers have gained useful experience and make a valuable contribution to social work in the community. The younger of such social workers are being seconded for general social work training and it is hoped that in time all local authority social workers will have taken an appropriate training.

CHILD CARE OFFICER

The local authority, through its children's officer and his staff of child care officers, is responsible for the welfare of children deprived of a normal home life (see page 132). The child care officer may supervise a child in his own home or, at the request of a parent or on instruction from a court, may take a child 'into care'. This places the children's officer in loco parentis and he becomes in law responsible for the child. The child may then be admitted to a residential children's home or boarded out with approved and registered foster parents where his progress is supervised by the child care officer.

The child care officer is sometimes a professionally trained caseworker who has followed one of the courses of training described on page 94. Others have taken a shorter training rather similar to that of the general social worker: while others are untrained, some with considerable experience similar to their colleagues in the health and welfare services of the local authority. In 1964, of the 1773 whole time child care officers in England and Wales, 28 per cent had the 'letter of recognition' from the Home Office recognising their status as trained or suitably experienced social workers: 32 per cent had a degree or diploma in social science and the remaining 40 per cent were untrained. The training of child care officers comes under the general supervision of the Home Office as does the functioning of a children's department.

PROBATION OFFICER

The aim of the probation service is to assist the social rehabilitation of an offender while he remains at work or at school under the supervision of a probation officer. It is considered that this is often a more constructive method of dealing with an offender than sentencing him to a period of imprisonment or imposing a fine. Most probation orders are conditional in that they require the offender to report regularly to the probation officer and to be of good behaviour; and may require him to live in a specific place, e.g. a boys' hostel. If the terms of the probation order are infringed, the offender is brought again before the court and receives the appropriate sentence for the original offence.

In addition to his responsibility to 'advise, assist and befriend' children and adults who are put on probation, the probation officer is available to give help in cases of marital difficulty. He may try to effect a reconciliation at the request of one of the partners and to give them support during this transition period. Should it be necessary, he can give advice how a legal separation and maintenance order may be obtained or how to start divorce proceedings.

Every magistrate's court and superior criminal court has probation officers of both sexes. A proportion are professionally trained caseworkers: others have taken shorter social science and social work courses approved by the Home Office while some have had in-service training only.

FAMILY CASEWORKER

The family caseworker is usually employed by one of several voluntary organisations which are still pioneering new services and filling gaps in the statutory social services. The principal organisations are the Family Welfare Association which, as the Charity Organisation Society, pioneered casework in the nineteenth century; and the Family Service Units which developed from the Service Units founded by the Society of Friends during the Second World War, in which many conscientious objectors gave help to evacuated families and victims of air raids. These caseworkers especially help families in danger of breakdown through illness, debt or other severe social difficulty and the Family Service Units in particular concentrate on the so-called 'problem families'. These are families with a multiplicity of problems who tend to show a number of common characteristics: the parents are often of fairly low intelligence or suffer from chronic illness, the father is frequently unemployed, the mother is often a 'bad manager' and runs into arrears with the rent, they have large families of children one or more of whom may be a delinquent. These families do not consider themselves to be 'problems' but are labelled as such by society; a more accurate and kinder term would be 'families with problems'. A few local authorities are appointing family caseworkers especially to help such families, another example of a service pioneered by voluntary organisations and now recognised by and incorporated into the statutory services.

The Family Discussion Bureau is another voluntary organisation whose main function is to help married couples with problems of adjustment and sexual relationships. Because the methods used by these caseworkers rely heavily on dynamic psychology, they may be of greater help to the more articulate couples. In this connection it is important to emphasise that the caseworker is not a psychotherapist: although both utilise the same theories, their aims and methods are different. 'The social caseworker's role would appear to be more active and educational than that of the psychotherapist. Her aim is more limited and is concerned with changing attitudes rather than with the personality.' (Lloyd-Davis, 1958, p. 43.)

MORAL WELFARE WORKER

These social workers, who are all women, are concerned with the problems arising from unmarried parenthood. Although the local authority is statutorily responsible for the health and welfare of unmarried mothers and their children, there is so much public apathy about their difficulties that few local authorities have developed services and the majority subsidise voluntary organisations and delegate their statutory duties to them. This is a field in which religious organisations have for long been active and most of the major religions and denominations have their own organisations. The largest is Welcare run by the Church of England through its Board of Social Responsibility. It has trained caseworkers (many of whom have taken a specialised training run in conjunction with Liverpool University) in all areas of Great Britain who, in addition to helping members of the Church of England, will give casework help to any woman in the absence of a co-religionist social worker or to women of no religious persuasion. The organisation runs homes for the care of women during the latter part of their pregnancies and for the care of mothers and babies for a few weeks after birth while the women are deciding their future plans. (Hall and Howes, 1965.)

Reference has already been made to the change in attitude that has occurred among social workers over the last fifty years and it is very marked in this field. The women and girls, some of whom are school children, are given the specialised help they require with their practical and emotional problems. A more recent development is the offer of help to the unmarried father whose own practical and emotional difficulties are usually overlooked but which may be quite severe.

VOLUNTARY SOCIAL WORKERS

A number of social services are staffed by unpaid and usually untrained men and women together with some trained people who give their time and skill free. Each service is organised on a local basis and the volunteers are supervised by a salaried full-time administrator who is usually a trained social worker.

In London, the school care committees are an example of this type of organisation. Each school in the Inner London Education Authority area has a voluntary care committee worker who acts as a liaison officer between the school and the children's parents and the school medical service. The workers are supervised by a social worker on the staff of the local education authority.

London and nearly all large cities have Councils of Social Service. These provide a social work service to supplement that of the local health and welfare authority when required, usually at a more personal and less skilled level. Some have volunteers of sufficient skill to be able to provide a family casework service, particularly in areas where there is no branch of the Family Welfare Association or Family Service Unit.

Citizens' Advice Bureaux are voluntary organisations. There are approximately 500 in England and Wales, most of which are run in conjunction with the Family Welfare Association or with local Councils of Social Service. They are to varying extents financed by these voluntary organisations with subsidies from local authorities. Most are staffed by a nucleus of salaried social workers with full or part-time assistants who all have an in-service training. They provide an advisory service to the public on any aspect of social legislation or with personal problems. Sometimes they give all the necessary help themselves and other times refer the enquirer to an agency specialising in the particular problem. Most of their clients have marital problems or difficulties concerning landlord or tenant.

The last few years has seen an upsurge of voluntary effort in the community. Many church groups have started 'Good Neighbour' Schemes while Task Force has enlisted the energy and enthusiasm of young people.

9

THE HOSPITAL TEAM

MEDICAL PERSONNEL

The medical personnel with clinical responsibility for patients comprise the specialists in the different branches of medicine and surgery and their supporting teams of registrars and house officers. Departments providing specialist services by medically qualified personnel include the various branches of pathology, diagnostic radiology and anaesthetics. In the community the general practitioner occupies the key position in the patient's care: in hospital this role is held by the clinician having clinical responsibility for the patient.

NURSING PERSONNEL

Of the non-medical personnel in a hospital, nurses have the most contact with patients, both in the outpatient clinics and in the wards. Increasingly, the role of the nurse in patient care has been analysed and its importance recognised. Routine nursing procedures offer the opportunity for influencing the patient's attitude towards his illness and treatment, thereby enabling him to receive greater benefit. In addition the nurse has an important function in maintaining the morale of a ward and in many instances becomes part of a therapeutic community. This form of treatment is in increasing use in psychiatric wards where all the personnel have a clearly defined role in psychiatric therapy in addition to their specific professional contribution.

PARAMEDICAL PERSONNEL

THE RADIOGRAPHER

The radiographer is professionally trained to work under medically qualified personnel in diagnostic radiography or in radiotherapy.

THE PHYSIOTHERAPIST

The physiotherapist works under the supervision of a consultant in physical medicine, an orthopaedic surgeon or other specialist. His or her function is to increase the patient's physical activity to its limit by appropriate active or passive movements and a variety of physical treatments.

THE OCCUPATIONAL THERAPIST

The occupational therapist also usually works under the supervision of a consultant in physical medicine or orthopaedics. Her contribution to the patient's rehabilitation is made in three ways. By providing him with suitable activities, she encourages him to use those limbs or groups of muscles that the physiotherapist has identified as needing continued development: the fact that the patient is, for example, doing weaving or using a fretsaw provides him with a satisfying activity that enables him to continue the required physical activity with less boredom than if he were doing only exercises. The satisfaction gained from creative activity is often an important part of treatment of psychiatric patients and cooperation between patients in the occupational therapy department can help an isolated or withdrawn person to mix more freely with others. Thirdly, the occupational therapist assesses the patient's ability to care for himself, whether he can wash, attend to his toilet, dress, feed himself and prepare and cook a meal. His independence may be increased by the use of appropriate gadgets or 'aids to daily living', some of which are standard while others may be designed especially to meet the patient's particular needs. The selection or design of the needed aids is assessed by the occupational therapist and the aids are often manufactured by other patients as part of their occupational therapy, or in the case of complicated aids by a technician attached to the department. It can be seen that the function of the occupational therapist and the physiotherapist are complementary.

Diversional therapy is the term used to describe handicrafts or activities undertaken by patients, not as a formal part of their treatment, but primarily to prevent boredom. This is important, especially in the case of long-term inpatients, as it keeps them active and interested and helps to prevent them from developing the apathy and dependence which characterises the 'institutionalised' patient.

THE SPEECH THERAPIST

The role of the speech therapist is twofold. She may give lessons to correct a speech disorder, such as stammering or lisping. She also helps to restore speech and the comprehension of speech in cases of brain damage such as that following a cerebrovascular accident. In these patients the ability to read and write may also be lost and have to be relearned. The speech therapist's first task is therefore to assess the patient's motor and receptive loss for the spoken and written word and then to institute the appropriate retraining. The occupational therapist cooperates by teaching the alphabet, reading or writing as required while the speech therapist concentrates on the verbal aspects of retraining. Because of the close coordination needed with the occupational therapist and physiotherapist, the speech therapist is often administratively attached to the department of physical medicine.

THE DIETITIAN

The dietitian not only supervises the preparation of special diets in the diet kitchen for inpatients but has a large educational role which also involves outpatients. Patients recommended a special diet by a doctor need to be told what they may and may not eat:

with certain diets patients may need special teaching in the methods of preparation. When giving such instruction the dietitian has to take into account the patient's financial circumstances and recommend ingredients which are within his means. She also has to consider the patient's cooking facilities as the preparation of a complex diet is easier on a modern cooker than over a gas ring on the hearth.

THE SOCIAL WORKER

The training and function of the medical and psychiatric social workers have already been described (see chapter 8, pages 95 and 98). It will be appreciated that the patient's care will be more smoothly integrated if the social worker also cooperates with all these personnel, as she often has knowledge of many aspects of the patient and his family that is relevant to the treatment they are giving. In many cases therefore the social worker occupies a central position, collaborating with the patient, his relatives, the medical and nursing staff and the other non-medical personnel.

10

THE MEDICAL AND SOCIAL SERVICES: AN HISTORICAL SURVEY

It is frequently implied that the welfare state was created in its entirety by one stroke in 1948. This is not so. The present provisions for the health and welfare of the population are the culmination of slow and often hotly debated developments during four centuries although the changes have been more rapid during the last fifty years.

During the centuries the prime responsibility for the provision of services has rested successively with the Church, with private philanthropy and with the community as a whole.

HOSPITALS AND SOCIAL SECURITY

In the Middle Ages, the monastic orders cared for the sick and the poor. There were about 800 monastic hospitals and those hospitals not controlled by a monastic order were religious communities largely staffed by priests with lay servants as in the monastic hospitals. While some hospitals were especially endowed for 'the maimed and sick' others cared for the aged and dying. The hospitals also helped the poor by distributing 'broken meats' and money at the monastery gates, the monk responsible for the distribution of these alms being known as the almoner. In London, two such hospitals were those of the Priory of St. Bartholomew in Smooth Field (now Smithfield) and of the Augustine monastery of St. Thomas Becket in the parish of St. Mary Overy, now Southwark Cathedral. With the dissolution of the monasteries by

Henry VIII the monastic hospitals were also closed, St. Bartholomew's in 1535 and St. Thomas' in 1540. The Lord Mayor and citizens of London petitioned Henry to refound the hospitals. St. Bartholomew's was refounded with a Master, four Chaplains and some nursing sisters in 1544 and in 1547 Henry re-endowed it, placing it under the supervision of the City. By the same Covenant, he gave the former hospital of St. Mary of Bethlehem (Bedlam) to the City as 'a hospital for distracted people'. During the reign of Edward VI the City of London purchased the Manor of Southwark and reopened the monastic hospital of St. Thomas the Martyr as the secular Hospital of St. Thomas the Apostle with 250 beds. For two centuries London was served by these three hospitals and there were few in the rest of the country. In 1713 Captain Coram established the Foundling Hospital to care for deserted children who otherwise died in the streets of London. Then in 1714, John Bellars, a Quaker, started his campaign for a hospital service to cover the sick poor throughout the country. With the cooperation of Henry Hoare a banker and Low Churchman and of three other men, public subscriptions were raised and the Westminster Infirmary was opened in Petty France, the first of the voluntary hospitals. The following years, Mr. Thomas Guy, a publisher and a governor of St. Thomas' Hospital, planned his 'annexe' for incurable patients who could not be admitted to St. Thomas'. 'Mr. Guy's Annexe' was opened in 1724 with 400 beds and subsequently admitted patients for treatment also, and remained an intergral part of the royal refoundation of St. Thomas' Hospital until 1825. 1730 saw the rebuilding of St. Bartholomew's by public subscription followed by the planned expansion of the Westminster. However, there was disagreement over the proposed new site and in 1733 the conflicting parties agreed to differ. The Westminster Hospital remained near the Abbey and a new hospital, St. George's, was opened with 250 beds in Landsborough House on the present site at Hyde Park Corner. In 1736 the Bristol Infirmary was founded and a hospital at Winchester: these two hospitals claim to be the first voluntary hospitals to be built outside London. In 1740 the surgeon Mr. John Harrison and four other gentlemen opened a subscription to build a hospital in the rapidly developing East End of London, the London Hospital. The Middlesex Hospital was opened five years later, at first mainly for maternity cases and Queen Charlotte's Lying-in-Hospital was founded for the same purpose. University College Hospital was founded in 1828 as the University Dispensary to provide clinical facilities for students of the Medical Faculty of the new University of London (later University College).

The effect of the dissolution of the monasteries on the care of the poor was as far-reaching as its effect on the care of the sick. The monks received pensions from Henry and many became beneficed clergy. The lay servants included young gentlemen of the squire class who worked as stewards and bailiffs but those of the domestic staff who were unable to obtain other work may have joined the ranks of the beggars. Some of the gentry who acquired the monastic buildings and turned them into manor houses continued the almoners' care for the poor at their gates but in general poverty was not relieved in this way. It has been said that 'the disendowment of the hospitals was more injurious to the poor than the disendowment of the monasteries. They had been founded to help the poor and had been placed where they were most needed.' Those who had begged for alms at the gates of the monastic hospitals had to turn elsewhere but there is no evidence that the numbers of beggars was appreciably greater after the dissolution than before. It has therefore been suggested that the system of almsgiving being 'unorganised and indiscriminate' did 'nearly as much to increase beggars as to relieve them'. It gradually came to be recognised that the provision of work for the unemployed and charity for the unfit was a responsibility not only for the Church and the charitable but for society as a whole. Under Henry VIII some towns, such as London and Ipswich, organised poor relief from the rates but in 1576, with the first Elizabethan Poor Law, England became the first of all European countries to develop a system of poor relief based on compulsory rates and discriminating between different types of indigent. The legislation was enforced by magistrates under the supervision of a vigilant Privy Council: in every parish overseers of the poor gave money to the unfit and bought materials to provide work for the able-bodied, while Houses of Correction were set up for vagabonds and those who refused to work. This Act formed the basis of poor relief for nearly two centuries until a new principle was introduced in the Workhouse Act of 1772, whereby an applicant could be refused relief if he refused to enter the workhouse. Ten years later this workhouse test was abolished and only the elderly, children and the sick poor were admitted, so that alongside the voluntary hospitals for the treatment of the sick and Mr. Guy's Annexe for the care of the chronic sick there were the workhouses to accommodate the destitute sick. Some fifty years later in 1834, the Poor Law Amendment Act reorganised poor relief under Poor Law Commissioners, combined parishes into larger Unions of parishes each with a Board of Guardians and reimposed the workhouse test. The conditions in the workhouse were made far worse than those that could be encountered in employment in order to provide a deterrent to the workshy. This policy caused much hardship and misery for the unfit and the genuine unemployed: it was against these conditions that Charles Dickens campaigned in *Oliver Twist*.

The next milestone in the relief of poverty which involved another new principle was reached in 1911 with the introduction of national insurance. Old age pensions, sickness and unemployment benefit for low-paid workers were payable to an individual as a right provided he had paid the required number of contributions under the national insurance scheme and met a number of other conditions. Meanwhile for those ineligible for national insurance benefits poor relief continued to be administered by the Boards of Guardians until in 1929 the local authorities (the county and county borough councils) were made responsible through their Public Assistance Committees. These two principles, the payment of benefits as a right following contributions to the national insurance funds and the payment of non-contributory allowances according to need, were retained when the national insurance and assistance provisions were reorganised in 1948. They are the basis of the current provisions for the relief of poverty under the aegis of the Department of Health and Social Security whose comprehensive provisions cover all ages and classes of the population.

It has been shown that between 1782 and 1834 the destitute sick were one of the main groups admitted to the workhouse. When the workhouse test was reimposed and relief was given only to those able people who were prepared to enter the workhouse, separate wards or blocks were set aside for the destitute sick as workhouse infirmaries. These developed also into special infirmaries for infectious illness, tuberculosis, epilepsy and insanity. In 1903 the Boards of Guardians were required to provide 'curative treatment' for the sick poor. When the Boards were abolished in 1929 and their poor relief duties taken over by the local authority Public Assistance Committees, the infirmaries were also taken over by the local authority Public Health Departments and new purpose-built hospitals were also erected. So there were the large voluntary general hospitals which often had a medical school attached and smaller voluntary specialised hospitals catering for special groups such as children or people with diseases of particular systems of the body: and there were the municipal hospitals, some of them the former workhouse infirmaries, providing treatment or accommodation for the destitute sick and people suffering from chronic illness, insanity or infectious diseases. Both types of hospital provided treatment for those who could not afford to pay for it, the voluntary hospitals as a charity, the municipal hospitals as a statutory requirement: but the standard of medical and nursing care was initially higher in the voluntary hospitals while some of the stigma of the workhouse infirmary still clung to the municipal hospitals.

With the introduction of the National Health Service in 1948 the voluntary and municipal hospitals were nationalised and came under the control of the Ministry of Health (now the Department of Health and Social Security). Those hospitals with medical schools attached were placed in a special position with Boards of Governors responsible direct to the Ministry of Health with the added duty of providing facilities for teaching and research: while the non-teaching hospitals had Hospital Management Committees responsible to the Ministry through Regional Hospital Boards.

The twenty years of the Health Service has seen a great levelling up of the hospital service, so that many former municipal hospitals are now providing medical care of a standard as high or in some cases higher than the former voluntary hospitals. The teaching hospitals are beginning to lose their exclusive lead in medicine and in London the numbers of patients referred to them is beginning to fall owing to competition from former municipal hospitals.

The last few years has seen the introduction of a new concept on which the overall hospital plan for England and Wales will be based, that of the district general hospital. Each of these hospitals will be responsible for providing the hospital services for a defined population and most of the teaching hospitals have already accepted district responsibilities. District hospitals will be large, 900 or more beds, and most of the specialities will be represented in each. However, Regional Centres will be developed in some district hospitals for certain of the more complex specialities, such as cardiac or neuro-surgery or renal dialysis, which must serve larger populations. This plan offers many medical and financial advantages but patients and their relatives may have considerable distances to travel, while the closing of smaller hospitals may provoke local opposition.

PUBLIC HEALTH

While these developments led to a national hospital service and provisions for comprehensive social security, others led to improvements in the public health. During the eighteenth century epidemics, particularly of smallpox, cholera and typhus, were rife. Housing conditions for most of the population were bad, with little light or ventilation and no sanitation. Refuse and dung were thrown into the streets from where they were washed into the canals and thence into the rivers which were used for drinking water. The science of preventive medicine started when doctors began to observe the clinical features of epidemics, the influence of environment, the paths of infection and the effect of weather and season on disease. Dr. Percival in Manchester formed a Voluntary

Board of Health which tried to prevent mortality, disease and crippling among the work-people in the newly developing industries. Others reduced the high rate of maternal and infant mortality and Jenner introduced vaccination. By 1800, as a result of these measures, the death rate no longer exceeded the birth rate.

However, during the first half of the nineteenth century, increased urbanisation and an increasing population caused an exacerbation of the difficulties and the mortality rate again exceeded the birth rate. During this period Dr. Southwood Smith assisted by Dr. James Philip Kay conducted medical and social surveys: these provided the information on which Dr. Edwin Chadwick, the secretary to the Poor Law Commissioners, and Lord Shaftesbury based their arguments in their life-long campaign to improve the state of the public health. As a result of their work the first Public Health Act was passed in 1848. This and later Acts set up administrative machinery under a Board (subsequently a Ministry) of Health to provide sewerage, street cleaning and a clean drinking water supply. With environmental reform under way, the second half of the century saw attention focused on what are now called the personal health services. The great importance of maternity and child welfare was recognised and the health visiting service was started by a voluntary organisation, the Manchester and Salford Ladies' Sanitary Reform Association. Charles Booth of the Salvation Army and B. Seebohm Rowntree conducted classical surveys in London and York: Beatrice and Sidney Webb campaigned for the different needs of different groups of underprivileged: Sir John Simon, a surgeon at St. Thomas' Hospital and a great medical officer of health for the City of London, and Dr. William Farr, the first statistician to the General Register Office, continued the work of Dr. Chadwick.

While these preventive medicine measures were continued and expanded during the first half of the twentieth century, provisions for treatment of the sick person outside hospital were developed. 'Poor Law doctors' were available to treat the destitute sick but, with the introduction of national insurance in 1911 for certain sections of the working population, the insured person could obtain free medical attention from a 'panel doctor' – a general practitioner who was paid from the insurance funds for his services to those insured people on his 'panel' or list. As these provisions did not cover dependants, the maternity and child welfare clinics were enlarged to care for children under five and pregnant women while the school medical and dental service was later developed to care for the child of school age. While the panel doctor service was part of the national insurance provisions, the preventive medicine measures, the maternity and child welfare services and the school medical and dental service were the responsibility of the local authority, i.e. the county or county borough council.

Therefore just before 1948 there already existed the three main strands of the National Health Service: the hospitals, voluntary and municipal, which were absorbed into one national service: the panel doctor service which was extended into the general practitioner or family doctor service for the whole population: and the local authority service with the prime emphasis on preventive medicine but having treatment responsibilities for certain groups.

It is this tripartite structure of the Health Service that has occasioned the most criticism by those who work in it. There are many situations in which the standard of medical care and welfare is reduced by administrative difficulties and this is one of the causes for such professional dissatisfaction as exists in the service. At the same time, administrative departmentalism increases the difficulty experienced by different sections and different professional personnel in learning and understanding each other's role and this in turn reduces the chances of cooperative and coordinated action. This situation has been clearly demonstrated in several sociological studies, for example that by Jefferys (1965). There have been many ministerial exhortations for cooperation and in some areas this has been fostered, mainly by good personal relations between the senior personnel concerned, but it is now widely considered that administrative reorganisation is urgently needed.

The Medical Services Review Committee (the Porritt Committee) which reported in 1962 recommended the creation of Area Boards each with the responsibility for the three combined branches of the service.

In July 1968, the Department of Health published its 'Green Paper' containing proposals for the reorganisation of the administration of the National Health Service and invited comment. It suggested the creation of 40 Area Boards each consisting of about 16 members and having responsibility for the medical aspects of the three branches of the service, leaving the social services with the local authorities. Simultaneously, the Seebohm Committee on the Local Authority Personal Social Services reported. The two social work departments of the local authorities are the welfare department and the children's department. The social work responsibilities of the departments of health, education and housing are secondary to the main activities of these departments. The Committee recommended that these social work responsibilities should be transferred from these three departments and combined with the duties of the welfare and children's departments to create one unified social service department. They recommended also that there should be no administrative specialisation of type of social work within the new department and that as far as possible there should be no functional specialisation by social workers. The principle is that there should be one social worker available to help all members of a family, whatever the nature of the social problem and whatever the age of the family members needing help. The emphasis is therefore on the person or family needing help rather than on the kind of social problem with which the person or family needs help. The advantages to the person and family are that any request for social work help would be made to one department, whatever the help needed, and that the number of social workers concurrently helping a family would be reduced. These recommendations have been widely welcomed by social workers but deplored by many of the medical profession who do not want the social work services to be separated from the medical services of the public health department. However, the Seebohm Committee reported that they found no evidence that any better social work service was provided by those authorities in which the health and welfare departments were combined under the medical officer of health compared with the services provided by the majority of authorities in which they are separate.

In 1969 the Royal Commission on Local Government in England and Wales reported (The Redcliffe–Maud Report). Their principal recommendations were the creation of only sixty-one local government areas outside London, grouped in eight provinces each with a representative provincial council. The creation of few and larger local government areas raises the possibility that the principal administrative areas of the reorganised National Health Service might be co-terminous and as this book goes to press a revised 'Green Paper' from the Department of Health is awaited, which is expected to take account of the Seebohm and Redcliffe–Maud proposals.

HOUSING

It has been shown that provisions for medical care and the relief of poverty developed simultaneously and that the importance of preventive measures was recognised in raising the standard of the public health. An important influence on the state of health of a population is its standard of housing. The influx of unskilled labour into the towns during and after the Industrial Revolution led to the building of cheap insanitary houses, such as the back-to-back slum property of northern cities, and to accommodation in which the occupational requirements of the home-workers took precedence over their domestic needs, as with the cellar dwellers of Liverpool where spinning required a damp atmosphere. Associated with the sanitary reforms of the nineteenth century were the beginnings of government action over the provision of housing. Legislation in the nineteenth century developed along two lines. Housing was mainly built for private gain, with the exception of that built by philanthropic employers such as Wilfred Owen and by charitable bodies like the Guinness and Peabody Trusts. Government intervention first set minimum standards of structural soundness and sanitation, and following the Public Health

Act of 1875 local authorities throughout England could make by-laws controlling building standards.

As the standard of slum property deteriorated it became unfit for human habitation so that by the latter part of the century the need was recognised for a programme of slum clearance followed by the rehousing of the inhabitants; a policy which was subsequently authorised by government legislation but only sporadically implemented by the local authorities as the cost fell solely on the rates. The next stage of development of a housing policy therefore was the introduction during the twentieth century of exchequer subsidies for programmes of slum clearance and new building, the basic rate of subsidy payable being dependent on the needs and resources of the local authority. Such local authority property is usually let at a rent well below the 'economic' rent: some authorities have consequently introduced a policy of rent 'rebates' or differential rents whereby an 'economic' rent is set but tenants pay a sum which is related to their income rather than to the value of the property. However, this policy has now become a political issue and it is administratively difficult and expensive to operate.

While the statutory authorities were primarily concerned with environmental living conditions attention was also paid to the quality of life lived by the residents. In 1864 Octavia Hill laid the foundations of good housing management and her policy, still followed by the Society of Housing Managers, rests on three principles: that the landlord and tenant have a mutual responsibility towards the property: that the social and business aspects of housing management should be combined by having a trained social worker as a rent collector: that good relations should be maintained between landlord and tenant. The second principle causes controversy now that there is a higher standard of living and of literacy among working class tenants than there was a hundred years ago. Some housing authorities consider that the functions of rent collector and social worker should be vested in different people: while others consider that the rent collector's right of access and entry for acceptable administrative purposes enables him or her to offer social work help to those tenants who need it without making any overt distinction between 'good' and 'bad' tenants, and it can be offered by a person already known and trusted by the tenant. However, all agree that a small proportion of tenants need social work help in running a home and budgeting and with personal problems that may be manifest as rent arrears, so that most housing authorities have a welfare worker available to help when needed.

Another social problem of housing management today is the effect on people of being rehoused into new estates or new towns away from relatives and former neighbours and friends. Not only does this policy break up existing communities but it seldom offers constructive help in the establishment of a new community in the new area. This problem has attracted the attention of sociologists and physicians who have studied the changes in personal and social relationships and their social and medical effects (see Chapter 6). There is some evidence that mild psychological illness is more prevalent under these conditions and in the new high-rise blocks of flats, but as yet most housing authorities have paid little attention to the problems they may be creating.

EDUCATION

Another influence on the public health is the standard of education of the population. In the Middle Ages schools were attached to monasteries and chantries but with the dissolution of the monasteries the funds of these and other endowed schools were appropriated. During the Reformation rich patrons founded schools and in the late eighteenth century religious bodies set up charity schools. The early nineteenth century saw the formation of the National Society for Promoting the Education of the Poor in the Principles of the Established Church and the British and Foreign Schools Society. The work of these two societies in the opening and running of schools for the poor was extended in 1833 by the first grant of money by parliament for educational purposes: a grant of £20,000 was allocated for the erection of school buildings provided that the two societies could raise a similar sum by voluntary subscription. Towards the end of the century the opinion was gaining ground that education should not be left solely in the hands of the Church so that, in 1870, the Elementary Education Bill was passed which established School Boards to erect and run 'Board' schools. So there was the parallel development of state and voluntary schools. In 1902, with the Balfour Education Act, the School Boards were abolished and their responsibilities vested in the local authorities, who were required to provide secondary as well as elementary education. The Butler Education Act of 1944, on which the current educational provisions are based, states: 'the statutory system of public education shall be organised in three progressive stages, to be known as primary education, secondary education, and further education: and it shall be the duty of the local education authority for every area, so far as their powers extend, to contribute towards the spiritual, moral, mental and physical development of the community by securing that efficient education throughout those stages shall be available to meet the needs of the population of their area.' Over 90 per cent of the children between the ages of five and fifteen years in Britain are attending schools which are publicly maintained or assisted by grants from public funds.

One way in which the local education authorities contribute towards the 'mental and physical development of the community' is by the provision of special educational facilities for children who are educationally subnormal or who are suffering from physical disabilities or who are emotionally maladjusted. In fulfilling this responsibility, the educational and medical services of the local authority cooperate to ensure that the affected child receives the education most appropriate to his intellectual ability and his physical and emotional needs. In addition, the local education authority provides 'day release' classes for adolescents who have started work and evening classes for employed adults. These may be vocational courses leading to professional or technical qualifications or courses in a wide range of recreational activities.

Thus over the centuries the community has gradually assumed the prime responsibility for providing medical care, social security, education, accommodation and sanitary environmental conditions. Implicit in these developments is the philosophy that the community is responsible for the well-being of its members. For this reason Lord Beveridge's term 'the Welfare Society' is more apposite than the more popular 'Welfare State'.

These developments have not taken place without some strenuous and vocal opposition to the implicit principle and there have always been those who have abused the existing provisions, thus giving cause for complaint by the critics. Writing about 1550 Robert Crowley shows the abuse of alms-giving:

'I heard two beggars that under an hedge sate,
Who did with long talk their matters debate.
They had both sore legs most loathsome to see,
All red from the foot well most to the knee.
"My leg," quothe the one, "I thank God is fair."
So is mine," quothe the other, "in a cold air,
For then it looketh raw and as red as any blood,
I would not have it healed for any world's good.
No man would pity me but for my sore leg,
Wherefore if I were whole I might in vain beg.
I should be constrained to labour and sweat,
And perhaps sometimes with scourges be beat." '

In 1698 some rate-payers and employers were loud in their complaints about the Poor Law and one critic wrote that 'persons once receiving outdoor relief refuse ever to work and seldom drink other than the strongest ale-house beer, or eat any bread save what is made of the finest wheat flour'.

The prevention of abuse today by a small minority creates an administrative problem and also raises a moral issue: how much abuse is the community prepared to tolerate in order that the exclusive regulations do not also exclude those in genuine need? This dilemma applies to the availability of professional services as much as to the provisions of monetary benefits. There is no consensus of opinion.

PART IV
REFERENCE SECTION

11

THE MEDICAL AND SOCIAL SERVICES TODAY

In the preface to the fourth edition of 'The Social Services of Modern England' the author, Penelope Hall, compared herself with Alice through the Looking Glass, running fast to remain in the same place, so quickly does modern social legislation change. In the following sections, therefore, only the broad principles of current legislation are described, trends are indicated and readers are referred to the principal officers from whom details of services may be obtained for a particular area.

In these sections, the focus of attention is on the different groups of patients who may need special services rather than on the services which different statutory and voluntary bodies provide: on the functions and availability of services rather than on the legislative framework within which they operate.

ADMINISTRATION

The Central Government Departments mainly concerned with the medical and social services are the Department of Health and Social Security (formerly the separate Ministry of Health, the Ministry of Pensions and National Insurance and the National Assistance Board); the Department of Employment and Productivity (formerly the Ministry of Labour); the Department of Education and Science (formerly the Ministry of Education); the Ministry of House and Local Government; and the Home Office.

Many duties are delegated by Central Government Departments to local authorities. A local authority is therefore referred to as a local health authority if it has functions in the field of health: as a local education authority if it has duties in providing educational services, etc. The structure of local government is complex but streamlining is expected as a result of the recently published Redcliffe–Maud Report on Local Government. For most areas in England and Wales the county council is the body responsible for providing the various medical and social services that come under the jurisdiction of the local authority. A borough council has certain duties in the field of public health and sometimes runs services delegated by the county council, for which the county council remains responsible. A county borough council fulfils the combined duties of a county council and a borough council. In London, the situation is unique. Since the reorganisation of London government, which became operative in 1965, each London borough has been the local authority for health, welfare and children. Each of the Outer London boroughs has been the local education authority but in the area covered by the thirteen Inner London boroughs a combined education authority has been established known as the Inner London Education Authority.

In any area, the clerk of the county council and of the borough council will provide details of the principal services provided by the respective councils and many authorities publish detailed brochures giving particulars of local services and amenities, together with the names and addresses of the principal officers. Where no printed information is available a written or telephone enquiry should be made direct to the principal officer at the appropriate county hall or town hall.

Services in Scotland and Northern Ireland are similar to those in England and Wales but the legislation and details of administration differ and are not described here.

MEDICAL TREATMENT

The Department of Health and Social Security is responsible for the provision of treatment through the three branches of the National Health Service. Primary medical care is given by family doctors or general practitioners. This service is organised on a local basis by an Executive Council. Each general practitioner has a 'list' of people registered with him for whom he is responsible for providing primary care and any person normally resident in this country is entitled to register. The general practitioner is paid though the Executive Council on a per capita basis, receiving a higher remuneration for older patients. Dental and ophthalmic services are also provided through the appropriate Executive Council. As patients do not register with a dentist or ophthalmic surgeon remuneration is by item of service.

Specialist consultation and outpatient and inpatient treatment are provided in England and Wales through fifteen Regional Hospital Boards and thirty-six Boards of Governors of undergraduate and postgraduate teaching hospitals, of which twenty-six are in London. Treatment is given through a variety of institutions: general and special hospitals: maternity accommodation: isolation hospitals and sanatoria: hospitals for the treatment of mental illness with accommodation for the care of insane and mentally subnormal adults and children: long-stay hospitals for the chronic sick: convalescent homes and medical rehabilitation centres. These are all secondary care services in that patients are referred by their primary physicians.

The local health authority, whose health duties are mainly in the field of preventive medicine, nevertheless provides medical care through its domiciliary midwifery service and its domiciliary nursing service.

All these major services are provided without charge to the patient at time of service. There is a proportionate charge for prescriptions with exemption provisions for certain categories of patient. There is also a proportionate charge for the provision of certain appliances such as spectacles, dentures and surgical shoes, but others such as calipers or wheel-chairs are free.

AFTER-CARE SERVICE

DOMICILIARY

The local health authority is responsible for maintaining the following services to augment the care of patients at home in conjunction with the general practitioner:

1. Home Nursing Service. No charge is made. (For particulars see p. 90.)

2. Home Help Service. This is a domestic help service financed by the local health authority (but often administered on a borough basis). The home helps are employed by the local authority to whom the patient contributes for the service according to his means.

3. Loan of nursing equipment, e.g. back rest, bed pan, commode, etc. Loans from the local health authority are free but these are often augmented by loans from the British Red Cross at a nominal weekly rental.

4. Many local health authorities provide a special laundry service for incontinent patients which is usually free.

5. Meals-on-Wheels Service. This is a service whereby a cooked meal is delivered midday to a patient unable to prepare one for himself and without others to prepare it for him. The local health authority is responsible for financing and organising the service but the local branch of the Women's Royal Voluntary Service often supplies the personnel to undertake the deliveries. The patient contributes according to his means.

6. The Health Visiting Service. The health visitors do not undertake any nursing duties but are available for health education, guidance and coordination. (For details see p. 91.)

The local welfare authority is responsible for augmenting the domiciliary care of physically handicapped or elderly people. Careful coordination of their services with those of the local health authority can greatly facilitate the home nursing or after-care of these patients. Relevant services are as follows:

1. Provision of gadgets or aids to daily living. These are special gadgets which replace or supplement a defective activity of the patient in order to increase his independence, e.g. a gadget to enable a patient with an immobile hip to put on his socks by himself: to enable a patient with arthritis of the shoulder to comb his hair: to assist a hemiplegic housewife to cook, etc.

2. Adaptations to the home. Structural alterations may be made to the patient's home (given the approval of the house-owner) such as installation of a ground floor lavatory, the widening of doors to enable passage of a wheel-chair, altering the height of the sink for a chair-bound housewife. Minor but often essential adaptations may be made such as the installation of grab rails in the lavatory or a monkey chain over the bed. Again, the aim is to reduce the patient's dependence on other people. For these services the patient contributes according to his means.

3. Recreational activities. Part of the success of good medical care is keeping the patient happy. The local welfare authority provides diversional therapy and other recreational and social activities for home-bound patients and for those who are able to go out to community centres and social clubs if special transport is available. For all these services the patient contributes according to his means.

4. As increasing numbers of patients have renal dialysis in their homes new problems of community care arise. It is necessary for the patient to reserve one room for the equipment which is supplied and maintained by the treating hospital and which requires special plumbing. Thus a patient may need rehousing and he may need structural alterations to be made to his accommodation. The housing and welfare departments of the local authority are therefore principally involved in this new form of domiciliary care.

For further details of provisions for physically handicapped people see pages 134, 136, 137, 144.

INSTITUTIONAL

Following a period of inpatient treatment a further period of institutional treatment of a different kind may be desirable:

1. Convalescent homes are run or financed by the Regional Hospital Boards to provide continuation of medical and nursing care in an environment where the patient can steadily increase his activity and independence before returning home. There is no charge to the patient.

2. Medical rehabilitation centres, which are usually residential, are run by the Regional Hospitals Boards and give an active programme including physiotherapy, remedial exercises and various kinds of occupationl therapy. There is no charge to the patient.

3. The local health authority may finance a so-called recuperative holiday when a patient has a medical need for rest, good food and a change of air and surroundings but is not in need of medical or nursing attention. These provisions are useful for the patient who is debilitated or who has been subjected to physical or emotional stress. Some local health authorities will use the provision as a preventive measure when a general practitioner considers that such a holiday would avert a medical or social breakdown. These holidays are taken in recognised recuperative holiday homes and the patient contributes according to his means.

CARE OF CHILDREN

Many services are provided by different statutory authorities for the benefit of children:

MATERNITY AND CHILD WELFARE

The local health authority maintains a number of infant welfare centres strategically placed in the community, from which the maternity and child welfare services are operated. These comprise antenatal clinics, a domiciliary midwifery service, well-baby clinics and immunisation clinics. The main purpose of the well-baby clinic is to screen the children for evidence of congenital or early acquired disease. Special attention is given to those children who are considered to be 'at risk' of developing an abnormality due to some complication during pregnancy or delivery. Such children are listed in the local authority's 'at risk' register.

There may be duplication with family doctors some of whom now run their own antenatal clinics, well-baby and immunisation clinics. They may hold them in the premises of the infant welfare centre, a policy which has the added advantage of improving the communication and cooperation between the general practitioners, health visitors and midwives.

The local health authority also provides, or assists voluntary organisations to provide, family planning clinics and a marriage guidance service often based in the infant welfare centre.

A free dental service is provided through the clinics for expectant mothers and children under five years.

DAY CARE OF CHILDREN

Day nurseries and play centres are run by the local health authority to care for children under the age of five years if their mothers are at work or are ill or during other emergencies. Priority for the limited places is given to children whose mothers are widowed, single or supporting the children herself, the 'unsupported' families: also if the woman is maintaining a chronically ill husband. Admission is arranged through the health visitors at the infant welfare clinic.

The local health authority is also responsible for maintaining a register of approved and inspected child minders or daily guardians. These are women, usually with young children of their own, who care for other people's children during the day in their own homes for payment. A scale of fees is recommended by the local authority but the final arrangements are made between the daily guardian and the mother. It is illegal to care for children for payment without being registered with the local authority. As there is a shortage of suitable daily guardians, children are sometimes placed by their mothers with unregistered women who, on inspection by the health visitor, deny that they are caring for gain and this is very difficult to disprove.

RESIDENTIAL CARE

The local children's authority is legally responsible for the well-being of children who are destitute or 'in need of care', for example if the parents are dead, neglected or ill. The social workers who carry out the authority's duties are the child care officers (see Part III, Chapter 8, p. 99). A child may be placed 'in care' through the juvenile court or at the request of the parents, for example if the mother is being admitted to hospital for so long a period that the father could not stay off work to look after him and when there are no relatives or friends available to do this. Attempts are always made by the child care officer to keep the child in his own home if possible. Some local health authorities employ specially trained home helps who will care for children at home before and after school while the father copes at night. When this is not possible, the child may be placed with a registered foster mother preferably in his home district so that he may keep in touch with his father and friends and continue at his own school if he is of school age. Foster parents are inspected and registered by the local children's authority and paid by them. If fostering is not possible or suitable, for example if the child is enuretic, he may be admitted to a children's home run by the local children's authority, or to one run by a voluntary organisation to whom the local authority pays the fees. For all these services the parents when possible make a payment to the local authority according to their means.

It is important to recognise that this scheme for the care of deprived children is separate from the remand homes or Borstals to which children may be sent as a punitive or preventive measure in cases of juvenile delinquency. Both schemes come under the aegis of the Home Office but their function and orientation are different. The child care officer is concerned with the child who is deprived of a normal home life and his duty is to provide a temporary or permanent substitute by using the local authority's various services. He is increasingly concerned nowadays with preventive social work, to offer skilled help to families at risk of social breakdown in order to avert a crisis and to avoid the child being taken into care. This kind of social work may also help to prevent the child from becoming a juvenile delinquent and coming before the juvenile court, not as being in need of care, but as an offender.

When he does come before the court as an offender he may come under the care of the probation officer (see p. 99). There is growing opinion in social work circles that the work of the child care officer and the children's probation officer should be amalgamated as they may be concerned with different children in the same family or with the same child at a different stage of his social career. This philosophy has been discussed in the White Paper 'Children in Trouble' and in the recent report of the Seebohm Committee on the Local Authority Personal Social Services.

EDUCATION

The local education authority is responsible for maintaining suitable day schools, and in a few cases boarding schools, for normal children from the age of five years to the minimum school-leaving age, at present fifteen years though this is extended in technical and grammar schools. (The minimum age will be raised to sixteen in 1972–3.)

'Special' schools, both day and residential, are run for handicapped children: the age of entry may be two years for deaf or blind children and the minimum leaving age for all is sixteen and often later. Separate schools are run for children who are blind, deaf, physically handicapped, emotionally maladjusted or educationally subnormal. The local education authority is in process of taking over from the local health authority the provision of training centres (in self care and minimum physical skills) for those children whose degree of mental subnormality renders them incapable of benefiting from formal educational provisions.

At special schools the curriculum and methods of teaching are adjusted to the medical condition and educational standards of each child and there is medical and nursing supervision. Application for admission to a special school is made by the recommendation of a medical practitioner to the principal school medical officer of the local education authority (see page 88) who makes the final decision whether or not to admit. This is a decision to be made with care. A child may benefit more from attending a normal school and mixing with fit children rather than feel he is being segregated with non-normal children. But special provisions at a normal school may not meet his needs and he may have difficulty in keeping up with his peers. Admission to a special school may remove this difficulty but engender feelings of apartness. The advantages and disadvantages of both forms of education for a particular child should therefore be considered very carefully by the child's medical adviser, his teachers, his parents and, when possible, the child himself before an approach is made to the local education authority: when the approach is made, it is sometimes helpful to make it in the form of a request for advice in the first instance.

When discussing special education for a physically handicapped child with his parents, it is essential to ensure that they understand the recommendation as parents often equate any form of special schooling with that for the mentally subnormal and react strongly against it.

In normal and special schools there is a free dental service. The medical service screens children at intervals, often at the ages of five, eleven and fifteen years: treatment is usually given by the child's family doctor or, in conjunction with him, at a hospital. If psychiatric treatment is required it is often given at the child guidance clinic of the school medical service.

PHYSICALLY HANDICAPPED PEOPLE

DOMICILIARY CARE

The local welfare authority has a general responsibility for the welfare of disabled people who are 'permanently and substantially handicapped'. This immediately raises the problem of definition of disability. Disability is best defined in functional terms as a limitation of performance of one or more defined essential activities of daily living in the areas of mobility, transfer, self-care, domestic duties and occupation. The concept of disability is thus distinct from that of impairment which is the anatomical, pathological or psychological disorder which may cause or be associated with disability. Thus every disabled person has an impairment but not every person with an impairment is disabled. However, each local welfare authority develops its own definition and hence its own criteria for determining whether an individual is eligible for its services. Furthermore, many of the provisions which the authority may make are permissive only, i.e. the authority is not obliged by law to provide the services but may use money from the rates and the exchequer to do so if it wishes. There is thus great variation in the kind and quality of services provided by different welfare authorities. People who are referred to the welfare authority and who are eligible for services have their names included in that authority's register of disabled people. However, these registers are incomplete for a variety of reasons: for example, the number of people referred is partly dependent on the availability and quality of services – the better the services the more will medical practitioners wish to use them for their patients: and the authority's criteria of eligibility partly controls the number of people registered.

The services which may be offered are of three kinds: provision of aids to daily living, structural adaptations to the home and diversional therapy. (For details see page 129.) People who need any of these services may also need one or more of the services provided by the local health authority (see page 128).

Employment services for disabled people are considered in the section on employment (see page 144).

INSTITUTIONAL CARE

Suitable institutional care is provided for different groups of disabled people by the local welfare authority, the Regional Hospital

Board and a variety of voluntary organisations. (For details see section on accommodation, page 148.)

CARE OF OLD PEOPLE

Cooperation between the general practitioner and the consultant geriatrician is often facilitated by domiciliary consultation. This enables the patient to be assessed in his home environment and suitable treatment to be planned.

DOMICILIARY

The home care of old people requires careful coordination of the domiciliary services already described (see pages 128 and 129). For this purpose many local authorities appoint special geriatric visitors: some are health visitors while others are social workers from the welfare department. However, if the recommendations of the Seebohm Report are implemented, many home care services of the health authority and all those from the welfare authority will be transferred to the new unified social service department, so that coordination will be simpler. A special chiropody service is now provided for old people by some authorities.

INSTITUTIONAL

The authority responsible for the institutional care of an elderly person is dependent on the extent of his need for medical and nursing care. (For details see section on long-stay accommodation, page 148.)

WELFARE OF BLIND PEOPLE

The local welfare authority has the statutory duty to maintain a register of blind people and the criteria for inclusion in the register are statutorily defined. An ophthalmic surgeon 'approved' for the purpose by the local health authority is required to notify the medical officer of health of patients meeting these criteria in order that registration and suitable services may be arranged. It is clear that the greatest tact is required when discussing proposed registration with a newly blind person: it is often best done by presenting it solely as an administrative procedure to inform the local authority as to who requires the needed service. Blind people may be helped in social and occupational rehabilitation through the blind welfare visitors and home teachers of the welfare authority. The Royal National Institute for the Blind runs social and industrial rehabilitation centres, while retraining and re-employment programmes may be arranged through the local welfare authority in conjunction with the Royal National Institute for the Blind and the disablement rehabilitation officers of the Department of Employment (page 144).

WELFARE OF DEAF PEOPLE

The needs of this group are liable to be overlooked as their disability receives very little public sympathy.

THE DEAF CHILD

Congenital deafness is one of the conditions for which babies are tested in the well-baby clinics (page 130) and it can be diagnosed at about six months of age. The greatest handicap of a child who is deaf from a very early age is the difficulty of acquiring intelligible speech even though he may learn to lip-read well. Communication remains his greatest problem and limits his employment chances throughout life. Early training is therefore essential. The baby can be fitted with a hearing aid in an audiometry unit of the National Health Service at about twelve months old and special speech and lip-reading lessons started at the same time. It is most important to teach the mother too, so that she may continue to teach the child throughout the day as a mother encourages any baby to talk.

The educational provisions for deaf children have been

described (page 133). Careful liaison between teachers, parents, youth employment officers (page 143) and prospective employers is essential and these services are often augmented by various voluntary organisations for the deaf.

THE DEAF ADULT

The local welfare authority has permissive powers to make provision for the welfare of adults deafened in later life after the acquisition of speech but these powers are used to varying extents by local authorities. The principal needs of the deafened adult are threefold:

1. He may need instruction in the efficient use of a hearing aid provided by an audiometry unit of the National Health Service.

2. In addition or alternatively he may need instruction and practice in lip-reading. Both kinds of classes are usually run by voluntary organisations, such as the Association for the Hard of Hearing, subsidised and supplemented to varying extents by the local welfare authority. Such training will often enable deafened adults to continue in employment. The elderly person suffering from nerve deafness cannot be greatly helped by a hearing aid and defective eyesight makes lip-reading difficult.

3. Isolation can therefore be a big problem: this may be combated to some extent by the social groups arranged by the voluntary organisations for the deaf and by utilising the welfare provisions for the elderly.

CARE OF MENTALLY DISORDERED PEOPLE

DOMICILIARY CARE

1. The local health authority is responsible for the domiciliary supervision and support of mentally ill people and their families, and trained social workers are increasingly being employed for this work. This authority also provides residential hostel accommodation for discharged patients and for chronically disabled mental

patients who do not need full hospital care but who need a protected environment.

2. The local education authority is in process of assuming responsibility for providing training centres for subnormal and chronic psychotic patients and for the day centres which provide custodial care and opportunities for socialisation. Its responsibility for providing special education for educationally subnormal children has already been mentioned (see page 133).

INSTITUTIONAL CARE

The Mental Health Act 1959 came into force in 1960. It swept away all previous legislation including the Lunacy, the Mental Treatment and the Mental Deficiency Acts. It recognises four types of disability: mental illness, subnormality, severe subnormality and psychopathic disorder.

Under this Act all admission of patients to hospital is normally on an informal basis in the same way that patients with physical illness are admitted to a general hospital without legal formality. When compulsion is necessary there must be a statement by a doctor that informal admission is unsuitable. A compulsory order may last for:

1. 3 days: an emergency admission for observation (Section 29).
2. 28 days: admission for observation (Section 25).
3. 1 year: admission for treatment (Section 26).

For the first order (1) one medical certificate is necessary together with an application for admission signed by a relative or mental welfare officer. For the other two orders (2 and 3) two medical certificates are required, one of which must be signed by a doctor 'approved' by the local health authority as having special experience in the diagnosis or treatment of mental disorder and it is desirable that the other should be signed by the patient's own general practitioner. These certificates must be accompanied by an application for admission signed by the next-of-kin or a mental welfare officer. If the next-of-kin objects to the making of a treatment order (3) permission must be obtained from the County Court for the application to proceed.

It is worth noting that a psychiatric patient may be admitted informally or compulsorily to any hospital, general or psychiatric, willing to receive him.

There are also powers of guardianship usually vested in the local health authority under which the guardian has the powers of a normal parent. These may be used to compel a patient, who no longer needs to be in a hospital but does require some supervision, to live in a specified place, for example a special hostel.

The mental welfare officer referred to above is a social worker of the local health authority. In the recent past he (or she) seldom had any formal training and his duties under the old Acts were largely administrative: but the changed philosophy of care embodied in the current Act has brought a change in the content and conduct of his work and this office is now held with increasing frequency by a trained social worker.

CARE OF UNMARRIED MOTHERS

The single woman often feels too frightened or guilty at finding herself pregnant to know how to ask for help and a doctor is often the first person to whom she brings her problem. During the pregnancy an unmarried mother will need help with one or more of three problems:

1. First, arrangements must be made for her to attend an antenatal clinic and to book for a hospital confinement. She may also need supervision and encouragement from a doctor or social worker to keep her clinic appointments regularly.

2. Her practical difficulties may include the problem of obtaining or keeping suitable employment with the related problem of financial difficulties. If she has paid her national insurance contributions she is eligible for weekly payments of unemployment or sickness benefit or, during the last weeks of pregnancy, the maternity benefit, and the lump sum maternity grant for the pur-

chase of the layette. Finding suitable accommodation is often a pressing problem.

3. Her emotional problems may include her relationships with the child's father and with her own parents.

Several social work agencies exist to cooperate with the doctor in the woman's care. The local welfare authority has the statutory duty to offer help from a social worker and to provide suitable hostel accommodation during the pregnancy. However, although people in general are now less censorious towards the single mother, there is general apathy over her welfare and few local authorities provide services themselves. This is an area in which religious organisations have for long been very active and most authorities prefer that they should so continue while the authorities fulfil their statutory duties by subsidising the organisations on a per capita basis. Most of the main religious denominations have a social work agency, of which the Church of England's Welcare is the largest with a social worker in each district (see page 102). If a co-religionist social worker is not available, the Church of England welfare worker will offer help to a woman of any religion or of none. The corresponding Roman Catholic organisation is the Crusade of Rescue. The various organisations run mother and baby homes which are hostels where the women may live during the latter part of pregnancy and for a few weeks after the birth of the babies while they decide their futures.

At this stage the difficulties may again be three-fold:

1. Financial difficulties may be acute. The child's father can be required by a Magistrate's Court to pay a maintenance allowance for the child if the mother applies for a paternity order but many women are loath to do this, some fearing that it will further decrease their chances of marriage to the father. The mother may claim the statutory benefits and allowances until she finds suitable work and can support herself and the child.

2. Accommodation is a pressing problem if she decides to keep her child. Some women take residential domestic work where she may have the child with her. Others find lodgings and place the baby in a day nursery or with a daily guardian: or some arrange for the baby to live with a foster mother.

3. The principal problem is the decision whether to keep the child or to place him for adoption.

Each of the main religious denominations has another social work section which is a registered adoption society and many local children's authorities have this function also. Every proposed adoption must by law be notified to the local children's authority by the person arranging it as the principal child care officer is guardian ad litem until the adoption is legalised. When the adoption is being arranged by a child care officer, the juvenile court appoints another social worker, often a probation officer, to be the guardian ad litem. It is the duty of this guardian to investigate the details of the proposed adoption, to report to the magistrates on its suitability and to supervise the adoptive parents during the 'probationary' period before the adoption is finalised. These arrangements have been developed to safeguard the interests of the mother, the child and the adoptive parents. Although it is legal for any member of the public, including doctors or nurses, to arrange adoptions the policy is much to be deprecated as they have not the facilities for making the necessary investigations even if they wished to do so. In an attempt to limit these 'third party' adoptions, there is much pressure from the organisations concerned for the passage of legislation requiring that the 'third party' should attend the court to present details and to be questioned by the magistrates.

CARE OF TUBERCULOUS PATIENTS

A doctor diagnosing a case of pulmonary tuberculosis is required to send the particulars to the medical officer of health of the borough. He notifies the physician in charge of the local authority's chest clinic which may be based in the chest department of a general hospital. The chest physician, health visitor and social workers are responsible for the out-patient treatment and welfare of notified cases of pulmonary tuberculosis and for tracing and checking contacts.

The Regional Hospital Board is responsible for providing

facilities for inpatient treatment. Because drug treatment is so effective patients are now usually admitted to general hospitals and many sanatoria have been closed.

CARE OF PATIENTS WITH VENEREAL DISEASE

Clinics for the treatment of patients suffering from sexually-transmitted disease are based in most general hospitals. No letter of referral from a medical practitioner is required and anyone may attend for examination and reassurance or for treatment. A special system of record-keeping enables all patients to be treated confidentially which is a matter of considerable importance. No charge is made for prescriptions. The tracing of contacts is a very important aspect of preventive medicine and is usually undertaken by health visitors working with the venereologist. A medical social worker is also available in the clinic to offer skilled help to patients, some of whom have severe emotional problems.

Following a decline in prevalence during the mid-1950's the numbers are now rising, particularly among young people under twenty-five years of age, homosexuals and immigrants. Most clinics have doubled, and some trebled, the annual number of new patients in the last ten years. More patients attend in large cities and nearly 50 per cent of all new cases in England and Wales attend clinics in the Greater London area.

EMPLOYMENT

EMPLOYMENT EXCHANGES

The Department of Employment and Productivity (formerly the Ministry of Labour) maintains at the local employment exchanges a register of people who are unemployed and available for work. The exchange also maintains lists of advertised vacancies which it aims to fill from the lists of unemployed people. Unemployment benefit is paid to them through the local exchange until they obtain suitable employment or until the expiry of their eligibility for benefit.

YOUTH EMPLOYMENT BUREAU

There is a separate Youth Employment Bureau for adolescents of fifteen to seventeen years, usually a special branch of the Department of Employment although some local education authorities provide this service. The youth employment officer maintains close contact with the school-leaver during his last term, with the head teacher, parents and prospective employers. After the adolescent has started work, the officer tries to maintain contact for up to three years.

REGISTERED DISABLED PEOPLE

Through the Disabled Person's Employment Act the Department has additional duties. It maintains a register of all disabled people who are considered to be employable and who wish to register, and whose application is backed by a medical certificate. The Department uses a functional definition of disability (see page 135): a person is considered to be eligible for registration as disabled if his disability is such that he is unable to obtain or hold employment in competition with fit people. The medical certificate, completed by the doctor who has treated the disabled person, requires a careful analysis of the man's residual abilities, comments on his mental and emotional state and details of environmental working conditions to be avoided. Each employment exchange has one official known as the disablement resettlement officer (the D.R.O.) whose special duty is to help registered disabled people obtain suitable employment within the limits set by their disability as described by the doctor in the medical certificate. The D.R.O. will also visit a patient in hospital or in the hospital's rehabilitation clinic when he can discuss details with the doctor, physiotherapist, social worker and other professional personnel.

Employers of more than twenty people are required to employ a 'quota' of registered disabled people and the quota is at present 3 per cent of the total payroll. The Department runs a number of residential and day industrial rehabilitation units (I.R.U.s) where people may spend a period of usually six weeks after accident or illness to become acclimatised to industrial working conditions again. No medical treatment is given as the emphasis is on employment rather than on illness. In addition, at these units a person's suitability for employment in alternative trades can be assessed when it is necessary on medical grounds for a man to change his type of work. Retraining can then be provided in a government training centre or financed by the Department of Employment in other suitable institutions, such as the Queen Elizabeth's Training College for the Disabled at Leatherhead which is a voluntary organisation, or at a technical college of the local education authority.

SHELTERED EMPLOYMENT

So-called sheltered employment can sometimes be arranged for severely disabled people in one of the Remploy factories. As these factories are subsidised by the Department of Employment the employees are not exposed to the production pressure of competitive industry and they are able to receive the wage for the job; as the jobs are usually unskilled or semi-skilled the rates of pay are low. Some sheltered employment is provided by the local welfare authority in conjunction with the Department of Employment.

HOME WORK

Paid employment for the home-bound person can sometimes be arranged through the D.R.O. and local employers although the facilities are limited and the wages are very low. Voluntary organisations are sometimes able to help home-bound people by supplying occupational therapy materials and marketing the goods produced. Few people are able to earn a living in this way but some are able to augment their benefits or pensions within the authorised limits.

SOCIAL SECURITY

STATUTORY ALLOWANCES

Statutory allowances are paid by the Social Security branch of the Department of Health and Social Security. Under the National Insurance Act 1946 the majority of adults between the ages of fifteen and sixty (women) and sixty-five (men) are required to pay a weekly contribution to the national insurance funds as employed persons, self-employed persons or non-employed persons (usually people of private means). Exceptions to these general rules include some married women who may opt out, students and those with a minimal income. Employers also contribute in respect of each of their employees. These contributions entitle the different categories of contributor to various cash allowances. These may include sickness, unemployment, industrial injury and maternity benefits, retirement and widow's pensions and grant towards funeral expenses.

Benefits and pensions may be augmented by the Department of Social Security with a supplementary allowance, formerly known as national assistance. The size of the allowance is dependent on assessment of the person's need by a member of the Department and certain medical requirements, such as a diabetic diet, are taken into consideration. Under certain specified circumstances it is permissible for a recipient to augment his benefit or pension by small earnings up to a specified maximum.

The family allowance in respect of the second and subsequent children under school leaving age is paid weekly to the mother. It is not dependent on insurance contributions or the income of the parents. At the time of writing there is some agitation to introduce the principle of selectivity and pay the allowance only to families in need.

VOLUNTARY FUNDS

The financial help available through statutory sources is not always adequate and in cases of emergency a loan or grant of money for a particular purpose, or help in kind, may be made by one of many voluntary agencies depending on the person's affiliations. Examples are the Benevolent Funds of the R.A.F. and the different regiments, British Railways, Civil Service and the Royal Medical Benevolent Fund.

ACCOMMODATION

HOUSING

Most county, county borough and some borough councils are local housing authorities and have a programme of slum clearance and a redevelopment programme for the building of residential accommodation. Each housing authority maintains a waiting-list of families who will automatically be eligible for rehousing when their area is redeveloped and also a list of families who wish to be rehoused from present accommodation not due for demolition. In the latter group, priority is assessed on a 'points' system, additional points being given, for example, in cases of overcrowding and poor sanitary condition of the premises. Ill-health, caused or aggravated by the living conditions, is also a relevant factor. It has already been shown (Part I, Chapter 5, page 25, and in Part II) that rehousing can be an important part of the patient's rehabilitation. In addition, patients often ask for a medical certificate to support their claim for rehousing. Such requests need very careful investigation before a decision to support the claim is made. There is a national shortage of housing and families often wait many years for their turn, so a policy of selection is at present necessary.

HOSTELS

Hostels of differing standards are run for professional and working men and women by local welfare authorities, the Church Army, the Salvation Army and many voluntary organisations such as the Women's Royal Voluntary Service and the Y.M. and Y.W.C.A.

LODGING HOUSES

There are usually lodging houses in the main cities for vagrant men. In London, the former Rowton Houses have been separately renamed to increase their individuality. These lodging houses were founded by Lord Rowton at the end of the last century to provide decent, cheap accommodation for working men who came to London to find work. They are now owned by a limited company. Some offer rough cubicle accommodation while others have series of reasonably furnished, lock-up bedrooms with handbasin and hot and cold water.

HOMELESS FAMILIES

The Department of Social Security is responsible for providing temporary accommodation for homeless people. Emergency accommodation is given in reception centres where the people's circumstances are investigated and their suitability for other kinds of accommodation assessed. Families which have become homeless following rent arrears and eviction may then be housed in property belonging to the local welfare authority on behalf of the Department of Social Security. This is usually old institutional-type property but attempts are being made to keep the family together as a unit and social workers try to help the father to get a job to maintain the family, to help the mother to budget and the family to become a functioning unit again. When this stage of social rehabilitation is progressing well, the family may be offered a self-contained flat in welfare authority property and, when they have demonstrated that they can function with minimum support from social workers, they may be rehoused by the local housing authority. This policy of social rehabilitation is adopted with the family having multiple problems which cannot be solved separately (see Case History Number 2).

LONG-STAY ACCOMMODATION

Long-stay accommodation is provided for elderly 'infirm' and for disabled and chronic sick people by a variety of statutory and voluntary bodies. The body to approach in any one case is primarily dependent on the extent of the person's need for medical and nursing care:

1. 'Part III' or 'Welfare' accommodation is provided by the local welfare authority under the provisions of Part III of the National Assistance Act, 1948. It is for those who 'through age or infirmity are not able to care for themselves and have no relatives to look after them'. The accommodation may be in small purpose-built old people's homes or in modernised large institutional-type buildings which are often inconvenient and impersonal. Each welfare authority sets its own criteria for admission but in general the residents are able to be out of bed all day, to dress themselves and attend to their toilet with a minimum of help and are continent. Some authorities admit people who are much more dependent to the 'infirm' wards of the large institutional-type homes. Residents pay fees according to their means.

2. 'Chronic sick' care is provided by the regional hospital boards for people who are in need of constant nursing and of medical supervision. The beds are usually in the chronic sick wards of the geriatric services, while senile patients are usually admitted to the older mental hospitals. Modern geriatric medicine is increasingly a programme of progressive patient care, whereby the old person moves from the acute wards through the assessment and rehabilitation stages and then home in the community with the continued support of the health and welfare services discussed earlier (pages 128 and 136). Some patients who cannot spend all day at home alone, can sleep there but spend the day in a day hospital while their families are at work. For these two groups the interdependence of hospital and local authority services is crucial. For those patients who cannot return to the community at all, hospital care in a chronic sick ward becomes necessary.

3. The responsibility of the regional hospital boards for the

chronic sick covers all age groups but in general the only health service beds available for the young chronic sick are in the wards of the geriatric services. Similarly the local welfare authorities seldom provide Part III accommodation specially for the young disabled person. It is the voluntary organisations which, by and large, meet these needs. Homes are provided by a variety of organisations. The best known is probably the Cheshire Foundation started by Group Captain Cheshire, V.C. after the Second World War. These homes admit residents up to the age of about forty years: they are run as homes not Homes and the residents have a large say in routine and policy. In the majority of cases the fees are paid by the resident's local welfare authority or the regional hospital board.

In this area of care the main problem is to determine which form of care is most appropriate for a patient and this is often difficult in border-line cases or when the patient's condition fluctuates. A less rigid policy with unified administration and less geographical separation of the different types of institution is needed and may be realised when the administration of the National Health Service is reorganised (see page 116).

VOLUNTARY ORGANISATIONS

Mention has been made on many occasions of voluntary organisations. These are of two kinds: those concerned with the welfare of a particular group of people according to the kind of service they require, e.g., the Cheshire Foundation and the needs of the young chronic sick for appropriate institutional care: and those organisations each concerned with the needs of people suffering a particular disease, e.g. the British Diabetic Association, the National Spastics Society or the Ileostomy Association. The purposes of these organisations include the following:

1. To provide an information service for the guidance of sufferers and professional workers. This may be achieved by providing a meeting place where patients and their relatives may learn from each other how to live with the disease, by publicity

programmes to educate the public in the needs of special groups of people, by the collection and dissemination of factual data about the conditions.

2. To pioneer the provision of new services not provided statutorily and to form a pressure group to remedy this need.

3. To collect public money to support medical and social research of benefit to the group of sufferers.

4. To provide grants of money or help in kind to relieve distress among sufferers.

5. To provide recreational and holiday facilities for those people precluded by their condition or circumstances from using the usual facilities.

These organisations usually employ a staff of professionally trained salaried workers. Local groups are often formed up and down the country by people who have a personal or philanthropic interest in the aims of the organisation: they help to run the local services and money-raising activities.

12

REFERENCES AND SUGGESTIONS FOR FURTHER READING

Publications referred to in the text are marked with an asterisk. *

Chapter 1 THE PATIENT

Balint, M. (1964). *The Doctor, the Patient and the Illness.* London, Tavistock Publications.

Bloom, S. W. (1963). *The Doctor and his Patient: a sociological interpretation.* New York. Russell Sage Foundation.

Brown, K. & Freeling, P. (1967). *The Doctor–Patient Relationship.* Edinburgh & London, Livingstone.

Cartwright, A. (1964). *Human Relations and Hospital Care.* London, Routledge & Kegan Paul.

Communications between Doctors, Nurses and Patients and Aspects of Human Relations in the Hospital Service. (1963). Ministry of Health Report. H.M.S.O.

Hinton, John. (1967). *Dying.* Harmondsworth, Penguin Books.

Jaco, E. G. ed. (1958). *Patients, Physicians and Illness.* A source Book in Behavioural Science and Medicine. Glencoe, Illinois. The Free Press.

Chapter 2 THE FAMILY

Bott, E. (1957). *Family and Social Network; roles, norms and external relationships in ordinary urban families.* London, Tavistock Publications.

Bowlby, J. (1953). *Child Care and the Growth of Love.* Harmondsworth, Penguin Books.

Bowlby, J. (1952). *Maternal Care and Mental Health.* W.H.O. Monograph No. 2. Geneva W.H.O.

Bowlby, J. et al. (1956). Effects of mother–child separation: a follow-up study. *Br. J. med. Psychol. 29.* 211.

Draper, E. (1965). *Birth Control in the Modern World.* Harmondsworth, Pelican.

Farber, B. (1960). *Family Organisation and Crisis.* Monograph Soc. Res. Child Dev. *25.* 75.

Goldberg, E. (1959). *Family Influences and Psychosomatic Illness.* London, Tavistock Publications.

Grad, J. & Sainsbury, P. (1963). Mental illness and the family. *Lancet i.* 544.

Newson, J. & Newson, E. (1965). *Patterns of Infant Care.* Harmondsworth, Pelican.

Newson, J. & Newson, E. (1968). *Four Years Old in an Urban Community.* London, Allen & Unwin.

Richardson, H. B. (1945). *Patients have Families.* New York. Harvard University Press.

Sears, R. R., Maccoby, E. E. & Lewin, H. (1957). *Patterns of Child Rearing.* Evanston, Illinois. Row, Peterson & Co.

Spence, J., Walton, W. S., Miller, F. J. W. & Court, S. D. M. (1954). *A Thousand Families in Newcastle-on-Tyne.* London, Oxford University Press.

Titmuss, R. M. (1968). *Women, Wife and Worker.* Problems of Progress in Industry No. 10. London. H.M.S.O.

Whiting, J. W. & Child, I. L. (1953). *Child Training & Personality: A Cross Cultural Study.* New Haven, Yale University Press.

Willmott, P. & Young, M. (1960). *Family and Class in a London Suburb.* London, Routledge & Kegan Paul.

Wimperis, V. (1960). *The Unmarried Mother and her Child.* London, Allen & Unwin.

Wynn, M. (1964). *Fatherless Families.* London, Michael Joseph.

Young, M. & Willmott, P. (1964). *Family and Kinship in East London.* Harmondsworth, Pelican.

Yudkin, S. & Holme, A. (1963). *Working Mothers and their Children*. London, Michael Joseph.

For additional studies of social and psychological effects of culture and environment see reading list for Chapter 6, Attitudes and Relationships.

Chapter 3 OCCUPATION

*Case, R. A. M. (1969). Some environmental carcinogens. *Proc. R. Soc. Med., 62,* 1061.

**Classification of Occupations* (1966). General Register Office. London. H.M.S.O.

*Dunn, J. P. and Cobb, S. (1962). Frequency of peptic ulcer among executives, craftsmen and foremen. *J. occup. Med., 4,* 343.

Hunter, D. (1968). *The Diseases of Occupations*. 4th Ed. London, English Universities Press.

*Morris, J. N. (1964). *Uses of Epidemiology*. 2nd Ed. Edinburgh & London, E. & S. Livingstone.

Schilling, R. S. F. (1960). *Modern Trends in Occupational Health*. London, Butterworth.

Chapter 4 FINANCE

Abel-Smith, B. & Townsend, P. (1965). *The Poor and the Poorest*. London, G. Bell & Sons.

A symposium on dietary habits of different groups. (1960). *Proc. Nutr. Soc.* Vol. *19*. No. 2. London. Oxford University Press.

**Employer's Sick Pay Schemes. Scope and Characteristics of.* (1964). London. H.M.S.O.

Hall, M. Penelope. (1963). *The Social Services of Modern England,* Chaps. 2, 3, 4. London, Routledge & Kegan Paul.

Nilson, B. (1964). *Cooking for Special Diets*. Harmondsworth, Penguin Books.

Chapter 5 HOUSING

Backett, E. M. (1965). *Domestic Accidents*. Public Health Papers No. 26. Geneva. W.H.O.

*Citizens' Advice Bureaux. *Report of the National Committee 1962–64*. London.

Hall, M. Penelope. (1963). *The Social Services of Modern England*, Chap. 7. London, Routledge & Kegan Paul.

For additional suggestions see reading list for Chapter 10, subsection on Housing.

Chapter 6 ATTITUDES AND RELATIONSHIPS

*Balint, M. (1964). *The Doctor, the Patient and the Illness*. London, Tavistock Publications.

Benedict, R. (1935). *Patterns of Culture*. London, Routledge & Kegan Paul.

*Bennett, A. E. & Garrad, J. Personal communication.

*Bernstein, B. (1958). Some sociological determinants of perception. An enquiry into sub-cultural differences. *Br. J. Sociol. 9*.2. 159.

(1959). A public language. Some sociological implications. *Br. J. Sociol. 10*.4. 311.

(1960). Language & social class. A research note. *Br. J. Sociol. 11*. 3. 271.

Brecher, R. & E. (1968). *Analysis of Human Sexual Responses*. London, Panther Books.

*Bronferbrenner, U. (1959). *Socialisation and Social Class* in *Readings in Social Psychology*. Ed. Maccoby, E. E., Newcombe, T. M. & Hartley, E. L. London, Methuen.

*Carstairs, G. M. (1963). *This Island Now*. London, Hogarth Press.

Drug Addiction. (1967). London, Office of Health Economics.

Drug Dependence. (1968). Home Office Advisory Committee on.

Hallucinogens Sub-committee. Cannabis Report (The Wootton Report). London, H.M.S.O.

Drug Dependence. (1969). W.H.O. Expert Committee on. Technical Report Series 407. 16th Report. Geneva. W.H.O.

Glass, D. V. Ed. (1954). *Social Mobility in Britain.* London, Routledge & Kegan Paul.

Hare, E. H. (1955). Mental illness & social class in Bristol. *Br. J. prev. soc. Med. 9* 191

(1956). Mental illness & social conditions in Bristol. *J. ment. Sci. 102. 349.*

Hoggart, R. (1957). *The Uses of Literacy; changing patterns in English mass culture.* London, Chatto & Windus.

*Hunt, P. Ed. (1966). *Stigma: the experience of disability.* London, Geoffrey Chapman.

Kluckhohn, C. & Murray, H. A. Eds. (1949). *Personality in Nature, Society and Culture.* London, Jonathan Cape.

*King, S. H. (1962). *Perceptions of Illness in Medical Practice.* New York, Russell Sage Foundation.

Lewis, A. (1953). Health as a social concept. *Br. J. Sociol. 4.* 109.

*Linton, R. (1956). *Culture and Mental Disorders.* Oxford, Blackwell.

Mead, M. (1950). *Male and Female: a study of the sexes in a changing world.* London, Gollancz.

Mechanic, D. (1965). The study of illness behaviour: some implications for medical practice. *Med. Care. 3* No. 1. 30.

*Merton, R. K. (1957). Revised ed. *Social Theory and Social Structure.* Glencoe, Illinois. The Free Press.

Merton, R. K., Reader, G. G. & Kendall, P. L. Eds. (1957). *The Student-Physician.* New York, Harvard University Press.

Miller, F. J. W., Court, S. D. M., Walton, W. S. & Knox, E. G. (1960). *Growing up in Newcastle-on-Tyne.* London, Oxford University Press.

Opie, I. & Opie, P. (1959). *The Lore and Language of School-children.* London, Oxford University Press.

*Parsons, T. (1951). *The Social System.* London, Routledge & Kegan Paul.

*Parsons, T. (1958). Ed. by Jaco, E. C. *Patients, Physicians and Illness*. Glencoe, Illinois. The Free Press.

Paton, W. D. M. (1968). Drug dependence. A socio-pharmolological assessment. *Advmt. Sci.* Dec. 200.

*Read, M. (1966). *Culture, Health & Disease*. London, Tavistock Publications.

Sainsbury, P. (1955). *Suicide in London: an ecological study.* London, Maudsley Monographs No. 1.

*Saphir, S. (1956). *Language, Culture and Personality.* California, University of California Press.

Schofield, M. (1965). *The Sexual Behaviour of Young People.* London, Longmans Green. (Also 1970 Harmondsworth, Pelican).

Spinley, B. M. (1953). *The Deprived and the Privileged; personality development in English society.* London, Routledge & Kegan Paul.

Sprott, W. J. H. (1958). *Human Groups*. Harmondsworth, Pelican.

Stengel, E. (1966). *Suicide and Attempted Suicide.* Harmondsworth, Pelican.

*Storr, A. (1960). *The Integrity of the Personality.* London, Heinemann.

Suicide, Prevention of (1968). Public Health Papers No. 35. Geneva. W.H.O.

*Susser, M. W. & Watson, W. (1962). *Sociology in Medicine.* London, Oxford University Press.

Wootton, Barbara. (1959). *Social Science and Social Pathology.* London, Allen & Unwin.

Hollingshead, A. B. & Redlich, F. C. (1958). *Social Class & Mental Illness*. London, Chapman & Hall.

Hollingshead, A. B., Ellis, R. & Kirby, E. (1954). Social Mobility and Mental Illness. *Am. Soc. Rev. 19*. 577.

*Querido, A. (1954) in World Medical Association. *Proceedings of the First World Conference on Medical Education*. London, Oxford University Press, p. 672.

For additional studies on the inter-relation of the individual and the family see reading list for Chapter 2, The Family. For additional studies of social and psychological effects of environment see reading list for Chapter 5, Housing.

Chapters 8 and 9 THE COMMUNITY TEAM AND THE HOSPITAL TEAM

General Practitioner

Cartright, A. (1967). *Patients and their Doctors: a study of general practice.* London, Routledge & Kegan Paul.

Collins, J. (1964). The Social work content of general medical services. In *Problems and Progress in Medical Care.* London, Oxford University Press. Nuffield Provincial Hospital Trust.

Field of Work of the Family Doctor. (1963). London, H.M.S.O. (The Annis Gillie Report).

**General Practice within the Health Service.* Report of the Committee on. Central Health Services Council. (1954). London, H.M.S.O.

Morrell, D. C. (1965). *The Art of General Practice.* Edinburgh & London, E. & S. Livingstone.

Nurses

*Butler, N. R. & Bonham, D. G. (1963). *Perinatal Mortality.* London & Edinburgh, E. & S. Livingstone.

**Health Visitors. Report of a Working Party on the Field of Work, Training and Recruitment of.* (1956). London, H.M.S.O. (The Jameson Report).

Stocks, M. (1960). *A Hundred Years of District Nursing.* London, Allen & Unwin.

Social Workers

Goldberg, E. M. (1966). *Welfare in the Community.* London, National Council for Social Service.

*Hall, M. Penelope. (1963). *The Social Services of Modern England*, Chaps. 8 and 9. London, Routledge & Kegan Paul.

*Hall, M. Penelope & Howes, I. V. (1965). *The Church in Social Work.* London, Routledge & Kegan Paul.

*Lloyd-Davies, A. B. (1958). *The Boundaries of Casework.* London, Association of Psychiatric Social Workers.

Social Workers in Local Authority Health & Welfare Departments, Report of the Ministry of Health Working Party on. (1959). London, H.M.S.O. (The Younghusband Report.)

Chapters 10 & 11 THE MEDICAL AND SOCIAL SERVICES

Hospitals

Abel-Smith, B. (1964). *The Hospitals. 1800–1948.* London, Heinemann.

Clark-Kennedy, A. E. (1962). *The London.* Vol. 1. London, Pitman Medical Publishing.

Clay, R. M. (1909). *The Mediaeval Hospitals of England.* London, Methuen.

McInnes, E. M. (1963). *St. Thomas' Hospital.* London, Allen & Unwin.

*Trevelyan, G. M. (1946). *English Social History.* London, Longmans, Green.

Tawney, R. H. (1938). *Religion and the Rise of Capitalism.* Harmondsworth, Pelican.

Public Health

Frazer, W. M. (1950). *History of English Public Health 1834–1939*. London, Baillière, Tindall & Cox.

Hammond, D. J. L. & Hammond, B. (1934). *The Bleak Age.* London, Longmans, Green.

Rowntree, B. Seebohm. (1901). *Poverty, A Study in Town Life.* London, Macmillan.

Webb, Beatrice. (1938). *My Apprenticeship.* Harmondsworth. Pelican. 2 Vols. (1948). *Our Partnership.* London, Longmans, Green.

Housing

Bell, E. Moberley. (1962). *Octavia Hill, a biography.* London, Constable.

Fanning, D. M. (1967). Families in flats. *Br. med. J. 4.* 382.

Hare, E. H. (1956). Mental illness & social conditions in Bristol. *J. ment. Sci. 102.* 349.

(1966). Mental health in new towns: what next? *J. psychosom. Res. 10*. 53.

Hall, M. Penelope. (1963). *Social Services of Modern England*, Chap. 7. London, Routledge & Kegan Paul.

Martin, F. M., Brotherston, J. H. F. & Chave, S. P. W. (1957). Incidence of neurosis in a new housing estate. *Br. J. prev. soc. Med. 11* 196.

Mogey, J. M. (1956). *Family & Neighbourhood: Two Studies in Oxford*. London, Oxford University Press.

Neighbourhood and Community (1954). University of Liverpool Press.

Taylor, Lord & Chave, S. (1964). *Mental Health & Environment*. London, Longmans, Green.

Young, M. & Willmott, P. (1964). *Family & Kinship in East London*. Harmondsworth, Pelican.

Children

**Children in Trouble*. (1968). Government White Paper. Cmd. 3601. London, H.M.S.O.

Clegg, A. & Megson, B. (1968). *Children in Distress*. Harmondsworth, Penguin Education Special.

Dent, H. C. (1961). *The Educational System of England & Wales*. University of London Press.

Donnison, D. V. (1954). *The Neglected Child and the Social Services*. Manchester University Press.

Douglas, J. W. B. & Blomfield, J. M. (1958). *Children Under Five*. London, Allen and Unwin.

Douglas, J. W. B. (1964). *The Home and the School*. London, MacGibbon & Kee. (1968 London, Panther Books).

Education in Britain. (1960). Central Office of Information. London, H.M.S.O.

Parker, R. A. (1969). *Decision in Child Care*. London, Allen and Unwin.

The Health of the School Child 1964 and 1965. The Report of the Chief Medical Officer of the Department of Education and Science (1966). London, H.M.S.O.

Physically Disabled People

Hall, M. Penelope. (1963). *Social Services of Modern England*, Chap. 19. London, Routledge & Kegan Paul.

Rehabilitation and Care of the Disabled in Britain. (1965). Central Office of Information. London, H.M.S.O.

Sussman, Marvin, B. Ed. (1965). *Sociology and Rehabilitation*. Washington. Amer. Sociolog. Assoc. & U.S. Dept. of Health, Educ. & Welfare.

Wright, B. A. (1960). *Physical Disability; a Psychological Approach*. New York, Harper & Row.

Mentally Disordered People

Caplan, G. (1961). *An Approach to Community Mental Health*. London, Tavistock Publications.

The Mentally Disordered. In *Health & Welfare: the development of community care*. (1963). London, H.M.S.O. Cmd. 1973.

Penrose, G. (1963). *The Biology of Mental Defect*. London, Sidgwick & Jackson.

Shepherd, M., Cooper, B., Brown, A. C. & Kalton, G. W. (1964). Minor mental illness in London. Some aspects of a general practice survey. *Br. med. J. ii* 1359.

Shepherd, M. & Davies, D. L. Eds. (1968). *Studies in General Psychiatry*. London, Oxford University Press.

Elderly People

Agate, J. (1963). *The Practice of Geriatrics*. London, Heinemann.

Bennett, A. E., Deane, M., Elliott, A. & Holland, W. W. (1968). Care of old people in residential homes. *Br. J. prev. soc. Med.* 22. No. 4. 193.

Harris, A. (1968). *Social Welfare for the Elderly*. Report of the Government Social Survey. London, H.M.S.O.

Hobson, W. & Pemberton, J. (1955). *The Health of the Elderly at Home: a medical, social & dietary study of elderly people living at home in Sheffield*. London, Butterworth.

Sheldon, J. H. (1948). *The Social Medicine of Old Age: a report of an enquiry in Wolverhampton*. London, Oxford University Press.

Townsend, P. (1957). *The Family Life of Old People: an enquiry in East London.* London, Routledge & Kegan Paul.

Townsend, P. (1962). *The Last Refuge; a survey of residential institutions and homes for the aged in England and Wales.* London, Routledge & Kegan Paul.

Townsend, P. & Wedderburn, D. (1965). *The Aged in the Welfare State:* the interim report of a survey of persons aged sixty-five and over in Great Britain, 1962 and 1963. London, G. Bell & Sons.

Administration and functioning

Anderson, J. A. D. (1965). *A New Look at Social Medicine.* London, Pitman Medical.

Bothwell, P. W. (1965). *A New Look at Preventive Medicine.* London, Pitman Medical.

Hall, M. Penelope. (1963). *Social Services of Modern England.* London, Routledge & Kegan Paul.

*Jefferys, Margot. (1965). *An Anatomy of Social Welfare Services.* London, Michael Joseph.

**Local Authority and Allied Personal Social Services.* (1968). London, H.M.S.O. (The Seebohm Report).

**Local Government in England.* (1969). Royal Commission. 1966–69. Vol. 1. Report Cmd. No. 4040. London H.M.S.O. Short version. (1969). *Local Government Reform.* Cmd. No. 4039. London, H.M.S.O. (The Redcliffe–Maud Report).

MacNalty, A. S. (1948). Medicine & the public health. *Br. med. J. ii.* 6.

McKeown, T. (1965). *Medicine in Modern Society.* London, Allen & Unwin.

*Medical Services Review Committee (1962). *A Review of the Medical Services In Great Britain. Social Assay.* London, H.M.S.O. (The Porritt Report.)

*National Health Service. (1968). *The Administrative Structure of the Medical & Related Services in England & Wales.* London, H.M.S.O. (The Green Paper.) 1970 2nd Ed.

Titmuss, R. M. (1963). *Essays on the Welfare State.* London, Unwin University Books. 2nd Ed.

Addendum

A posthumous edition of Hall's *Social Services of Modern England* has now been produced under the title *Penelope Hall's Social Services of England and Wales* (1969). Forder A., Ed. London, Routledge & Kegan Paul.

INDEX

Page numbers printed in bold type indicate main references